MW00633891

CHRONIC PAIN CONTROL

THIRD EDITION

CHRONIC PAIN CONTROL

ALTERING REALITY 3.0

INTRINSIC ALTERNATIVES
FOR PAIN MANAGEMENT

VICKI ELLIS

CREATING BALANCE PUBLISHING

First edition, October 2016
Second edition, May 2019
Third edition, May 2020

ISBN-13: 978-0-9972415-7-0

Book design by Vicki Ellis
Editing support with Sara M Janus
Head shot photo and logo illustrations by
Mike Barry at FortCollinsWebWorks.com
Cerebral Cortex Neuron cover illustration by Vicki Ellis

*This work is dedicated to those searching for
intrinsic ways to control their chronic pain,
and help prevent overexposure to opioids,
naturally and effectively, from within.*

CONTENTS

Part IV

Preface

Chronic Pain Control: Altering Reality 3.0 is for adults to learn how to control chronic and some acute pains from within, even to the point of stopping them. These skills are effective for most painful conditions, but we restrict their use to only control pains that are safe to control. For example, it could become life-threatening if we were to stop feeling pain from an infection too soon.

I've experienced chronic pain since 1960, having suffered from torn muscles, glands, ligaments, tendons, damaged joints, pinched spinal nerves and spinal cord, broken bones, and have had many surgeries over my lifetime. I controlled severe pain for a few moments back in 1977. After trying to repeat that through trial and error over the decades that followed, I finally succeeded in 2010.

I studied neurobiology to earn my master's degree in Anatomy/Biomedical Science (2001) and taught college biomedical science courses, including neurobiology. Not realizing it at the time, my education in neuroscience would help me teach you pain control many years later.

Once I figured out how to control my own chronic pain, it took time to fully develop those methods. By 2013, I began teaching others to successfully control their chronic pain, too. By 2014, my chronic pain was not just controlled, it was totally gone. My nervous system changed its relationship with pain entirely.

In 2015, one of my pain control students suggested I write a book to describe, preserve, and share my techniques. Thanks to her, I published my first chronic pain control book in 2016. Several editions followed as descriptions were rewritten with more clarity and completeness, the techniques were tested on more conditions, more discoveries were made, and more topics were added to the book, as the techniques evolved. I believe it is complete now. I'd like to help adult students learn more about pain and how to control it as effectively and SAFELY as possible.

Since 2014, I have collected hundreds of neuroscience journal articles, whose current research supports the validity of these techniques. A future chronic pain control book is planned to incorporate details from those articles. My neuroscience background, independent research from around the world, my personal, lifelong experience with pain, and successfully controlling it, plus student successes with their various painful conditions are critical factors that ensure this book offers effective techniques for learning how to control chronic pain. These techniques can minimize exposure to opioids and help prevent dependence and/or addiction.

The book has been divided into parts. The Table of Contents gives you a road map with descriptive topics for locating sections to reread and study, as you practice and improve your skills over time.

Part I provides the background story which lead to my discovering and further developing these pain control techniques. It also teaches, at a basic level, the neuroscience that relates to how the techniques work.

Part II gives instructions for correctly applying the CB Intrinsic® (CBi) Touch to the skin or hair for quickly controlling pain. Since it works from the injury site up to the brain, we call it bottom-up control over pain. Believing in it is not required for it to work, so we can also use it to help our furry pets that suffer from painful chronic conditions, such as arthritis.

Part III describes how and explains why ten CBi Mindfulness-based Pain Control (MBPC) techniques work. Directed from the brain down toward the body, they provide long-term, top-down control over pain. They utilize neuroplasticity, which allows the whole nervous system to unlearn abnormal, unnecessary chronic pain patterns. They teach us how to control stress, so it won't exacerbate our pain. MBPC helps in more ways than just pain control, and it can improve the quality of life and health of mind, body and spirit.

Part IV helps significant others, family members, friends, and practitioners, who cannot see or feel the pain, imagine what chronic pain is like to appreciate it more fully from someone else's perspective. Common issues are raised and solutions suggested to foster healthy, positive pain control partnerships for successful application of pain control techniques together.

Perhaps Part V should have been Part I because it teaches vital and crucial safety information. Precautions and Limitations addresses serious life-threatening dangers inherent in controlling pain. We prohibit controlling pain if that pain serves a vital purpose. We must always avoid causing further harm.

Pain hurts a lot, but it is our friend. It warns us of a full range of conditions, from minor scrapes to potentially life threatening conditions. Yet we can minimize suffering from pain that won't stop on its own, and/or that which no longer or never did serve a purpose. The CB Intrinsic Touch and Mindfulness-based Pain Control techniques minimize many of the ill effects caused by suffering from unnecessary pain.

Yes, This Actually Is Revolutionary.

Part I

ORIGINS OF CB INTRINSIC CHRONIC PAIN CONTROL

What a Pain

Depending on the study, it has been estimated that roughly 100 million American adults suffer from chronic or persistent pain. That is about one third of the total population of the United States (2017). It has also been estimated that 1.5 billion suffer from some form of chronic or persistent pain worldwide.[1] Accordingly, given that the global population is currently around 7.7 billion (2019), an estimated 20% of the human population experiences chronic pain.

Acute pain serves the vital purpose of alerting us to possible tissue damage or some other medical condition. Once the damage heals sufficiently, or we have taken care of the condition, we expect its acute pain to stop. The nervous system creates the state of acute pain for a purpose, and once that purpose is finished, the nervous system normally stops creating that acute pain.

Chronic or persistent pain exists when acute pain fails to cycle off properly. Chronic pain continues without purpose. Chronic pain is an abnormal pain state.

The terms chronic and persistent refer to abnormal pain that lasts at least 3 months after tissues have healed. Acute pain may occur chronically, and seem

[1] Global Industry Analysts, Inc. (2011) Global Pain Management Market to Reach US$60 Billion by 2015, According to a New Report by Global Industry Analysts, Inc. PDF available from http://www.prweb.com/pdf download/8052240.pdf [Accessed March 21, 2018].

like chronic pain because the medical condition itself is chronic, so the condition continually creates new acute pain. Persistent pain conditions occur because the nervous tissue itself has been injured or damaged, and pain continues long-term until that condition heals. Sometimes the nervous system spontaneously learns abnormal patterns for creating pain that neither points to an injury nor serves a known purpose. In addition to creating needless pain, sometimes the nervous system forgets how to stop pain that it normally would have.

Given the numerous possible causes, multiple ways for treating chronic pain, and a wide range of treatment outcomes, the topic of managing chronic pain is very complex.

I'd like to distinguish the term pain 'management' from pain 'control'. For the purposes of this book, pain 'management' relies on pharmaceuticals, medical devices, personnel, interventions, and/or procedures to manage a patient's chronic pain, for the patient. On the other hand, 'control' enables the patient to manipulate his or her own nervous system to reduce or stop their own chronic pain. Chronic pain control is for, by, and occurs within the patient. Pain control can stand on its own or be added to pain management regimens.

We could say pain management originates outside of the body, which makes pain management 'extrinsic' to the body and nervous system. On the other hand, pain control originates inside the patient's body and nervous system naturally, so pain control is 'intrinsic' to the body and nervous system. The definition of pain control in the context of this book is - *students of CB Intrinsic (CBi) Chronic Pain Control techniques actively and intrinsically reduce, stop, and/or prevent the creation of chronic pain by teaching their own nervous system to restore normal or nearly normal pain processes.*

CBi techniques work to improve the effectiveness of normal pain control pathways by inhibiting or limiting further use of the nervous system's abnormal, persistent pain creating pathways.

These intrinsic techniques foster well-being and can be learned fairly quickly for effective, long-term pain relief. With some painful conditions, the techniques even allow weakened muscles and glands to regain some or most of their function and begin working again within days to weeks.

For example, by making it hurt too much to move, pain restricts movement in order to help us avoid causing further damage. Sometimes muscle restriction is about more than our simply choosing to avoid the pain. Sometimes muscle movement may be restricted by the nervous system as a separate part of the pain process. We notice that when we are able to push through the pain to force some muscles to move, the muscles are not able to respond, despite our best efforts.

With intrinsic pain control techniques, whether they were restricted by our avoidance or their inability, muscles often begin working again after the pain has been removed. CBi pain relief itself is amazing, but freeing up muscle function or movement, too, is doubly amazing.

Whenever there is an underlying condition, reducing or stopping pain is not a cure. Until they are cured, conditions or injuries may threaten the body's ability to function. It is essential that bodies work. If function is lost, as in paralysis, regaining it is very difficult. Protecting function is more important than controlling pain. Also, when an injury is very serious, symptoms other than pain may include nausea and/or doubling-over. Pain control methods cannot prevent the occurrence of nausea or doubling-over. Those symptoms continue to send out warnings of very serious injury.

It is important to continue monitoring the progress of underlying conditions by tracking all symptoms, particularly changes in muscle or gland function. Depending on the condition, protecting and preserving function is always primary; controlling pain is secondary. Once it is safe to control pain, it may become primary.

Examination of findings from neuroscience research studies sheds light on how the nervous system processes pain and how the CB Intrinsic Touch (taught in Part II) works. Research descriptions about the ways various components of the nervous system are activated by opioids, and even by acupuncture needles, correlate well with the same components that are activated by the CB Intrinsic Touch. They work through the same sets of cells or 'neurons' in the pathways of the nervous system that are responsible for pain's creation and cessation.

Mindfulness techniques have been used to control pain for millennia, especially in the East. The techniques remain popular because they work so well, when applied correctly.

By correctly practicing CB Intrinsic Mindfulness-Based Pain Control (MBPC) techniques (taught in Part III) to overcome chronic pain, one also experiences positive changes in mental perspectives and emotions, while experiencing healthy sensations throughout the entire body. With this enhanced expression of well-being, targeted directly at the pain, painful perceptions diminish and may finally stop for periods of time (days, weeks, months, years). Overall health improves naturally, as a direct result.

Many Westerners are familiar with the term 'mindfulness', but few actually know how to reach the state of mind necessary for effective control of *even very serious* physical pain. Cognitive neuroscience research is ongoing to help understand why and how mindfulness techniques work; the research continues to uncover more and more facts for an ever-increasing understanding of the processes at work regarding pain perception.

For the mindfulness component of chronic pain control, give yourself permission to ignore your old beliefs or mindsets in exchange for the MBPC mindset; this is the effective and powerful state of mind that eventually turns chronic pain into a memory, and potentially restores near-normal pain processing, plus hopefully a gain-in-function for muscles and/or glands.

People with various painful conditions have successfully tried these techniques. Relief came for sharp, dull, achy, burning, intense, and pins-and-needles types of pain. We have learned of several conditions that can benefit from the CBi Touch and MBPC techniques, including, but not limited to cystic fibrosis, fibromyalgia, diabetes neuropathy, spinal nerve and cord pain, surgery recovery, neuropathic pain, arthritis, osteoarthritis, organ pain, torn ligaments and tendons, broken bone, migraine headache, sprains, strains, and interstitial cystitis.

While applying the CBi Touch and MBPC together over the years, the nervous system and the whole body can learn to stop creating chronic pain and return to normal patterns: appropriate acute pain with an injury now, followed by no acute pain as tissues heal. Individual results vary because individuals, injuries, conditions, and skill sets vary.

At the very least, these techniques support and improve outcomes for pain management. For example, while experiencing pain, some muscle activity may be restricted, therefore, feeling less pain potentially improves physical therapy performance, due to less muscle restriction for routines. Less pain, less muscle restriction, measurable gain-in-function, and increased range of motion tend to improve physical therapy compliance and help improve message therapy results.

Since most adults should be able to accomplish pain control intrinsically, naturally from within, the descriptions and instructions in this book will help those experiencing chronic or persistent pain learn how to control pain for themselves by using these techniques. Mastering these skills is transformational, as one transitions from being a person controlled by chronic pain into a person who is able to control chronic pain instead.

Perfecting the CBi Touch and MBPC skills takes practice, but success and improvement occur fairly quickly. While using the CBi Touch (or simply the Touch), novices can significantly reduce pain within a matter of minutes. Dedicated students know they have reached the Chronic Pain Control Master level once they can control pain rapidly and automatically, with the reduction in pain lasting for an extended period of time. They may notice that they feel and think about pain less often, that their muscles are less restricted, and realize they can accomplish more things than they could while they were suffering from pain. Quality of life improves dramatically.

Skills for chronic pain control improve over time, due to a process called 'neuroplasticity'. Neuroplasticity refers to the nervous system's ability to learn, as it adapts to new input. Neuroplasticity results in long-term change. To reset normal pain processes in the nervous system, practicing CBi techniques naturally and appropriately decrease the production of abnormal pain, in exchange for re-establishing normal pain-processing pathways.

This happens behind the scenes. No one needs to try harder to make neuroplasticity happen. It happens naturally and intrinsically during practice. If pain returns, these skills are applied to reduce the pain again. Repetition supports forward progress, so chronic pain becomes less intense, returns less often, and remains silent for longer periods of time, even becoming silent for years or perhaps permanently. But it is essential that we control pain prudently and intelligently.

Please do not use these techniques, and then ignore present needs. The book title is *Chronic Pain Control* precisely because it is best to not use these techniques with acute pain, but rather wait until acute pain has served its purpose. It is best to wait until a condition has been diagnosed or the pain has been specifically diagnosed as chronic or persistent by a doctor. Always seek a doctor's advice regarding the use of pain control.

The reason for having precautions is that allowing the feeling of pain is very important for survival. Pain alerts us to a medical condition, infection, disease, or injury. Pain helps us locate the problem and know how serious it is. Pain prompts us to get help. And when the pain lessens on its own, that is an indication the condition is healing.

Also, doctors depend on our descriptions of pain to accurately diagnose conditions. Applying the CBi Touch and MBPC techniques to stop acute pain before seeking a diagnosis would obviously make it more difficult for a doctor to correctly diagnose the condition.

If the injury or condition were not significant enough for a doctor's visit, would it be okay to apply these techniques to acute pain? Not necessarily.

A seemingly insignificant condition might not remain insignificant. An apparently minor cut or puncture wound could become infected. A headache might not be just a 'headache'.

It's beneficial to continue feeling acute pain until you know more about the condition. Whenever pain intensifies, that's an indication the condition is possibly becoming worse. At that point, perhaps this condition has become significant, which means it is necessary to seek a doctor's help after all. Had the acute pain been controlled, a worsening condition might have gone unnoticed, with regrettable results.

It is tempting to stop acute pain right away, but acute pain serves a vital purpose, and without it, we tend to forget about the condition. Even though it's a pain, it is best to allow acute pain to run its course, or to wait until a doctor says it is time to control the pain. Saving these techniques specifically for chronic pain, and not using them with purposeful acute pain is wise and prudent.

This book does not intend to replace, object to, compete or conflict with doctors' medical advice. Check with your doctor before using the techniques described in this book, if you think there might be a conflict. We do not want to create further harm.

Some types of prescription pain medication can upset the body's delicate balance, interfere with 'homeostasis', the natural biochemical balance bodies try to maintain. Opioids and other drugs taken long-term can negatively impact parts of the nervous system that we rely on for CBi techniques to work. Those drugs can also disrupt the delicate balance within many other cell types found in the digestive tract, liver, kidneys, and other organs, thus injuring them, too.

Short-term use of pain medications, such as during and for a short time following surgery, does not appear to hamper the effectiveness of CBi chronic pain control techniques very much, yet anesthesia can diminish the effectiveness of the techniques for a short period of time.

Long-term opioid use affects the effectiveness of these techniques for some people, but not for others. If there is a problem, once pain medication treatments are finished and the nervous system has had time to recover from their use, CBi techniques' effectiveness improves.

Further, this is 'Opioid Overexposure Prevention' because CBi techniques help prevent the need for initial or continued opioid exposure, and the associated risks. Long-term reliance on prescription painkillers or opioid treatments becomes less necessary or unnecessary. By applying pain control techniques correctly, drug addiction may be prevented.

In addition, naturally and intrinsically restoring the nervous system's abnormal chronic pain patterns back to normal acute pain patterns can be accomplished through practicing CBi techniques. Pain medications do not do that.

Persistent or chronic pain shapes our sense of reality and controls our internal world. Chronic pain seems tangible and physical, but it is neither. Chronic pain controls us only because the mind tricks us. To switch that around and gain control of pain, we need to expand our knowledge and beliefs about our internal world.

The bottom line from all of this is that for even the most intense and unrelenting pain, the successful application of CBi Touch and MBPC techniques can significantly reduce or stop that pain for varying periods of time, and sometimes permanently. Since the techniques work for most sources and types of pain, controlling pain this quickly and effectively can change lives for the better. Having control over pain changes our relationships not only with pain, but also with the self, others, and life in general.

Reflecting on my education in neuroscience, I realized that understanding how pain processing works helped me unlearn my strong, decades-old, ordinary beliefs. Those old beliefs were ensuring pain would continue to control me. Removing those old beliefs allowed me to first trust and then master pain control.

Understanding may help enhance others' success with these techniques. That is why I write this book in order to share this knowledge of intrinsic pain control with as many adults as possible to help reduce physical suffering in the World.

Chronic Pain Control: Altering Reality, 3.0 teaches how to train the same nervous system that creates chronic pain to effectively silence that pain instead. It is written for the estimated 1.5 billion sufferers of chronic pain worldwide, and their significant others, friends, caregivers, doctors, nurses, physical and massage therapists, etc., who are interested in learning CBi methods for effectively controlling chronic pain. This may help prevent overexposure to and potential abuse of opioids. Remember: only adult minds, perhaps 25 years and older, are sufficiently developed and mature enough to apply these techniques safely.

It's just a matter of learning how to apply CBi chronic pain control techniques correctly and safely. The impacts of these techniques are extraordinary and revolutionary.

The Long Journey

Ever since I was a child, I have had acute, persistent, and chronic pain. I have experienced mild, nagging discomfort all the way to extreme agony, including trigeminal nerve, spinal nerve, and spinal cord pains. As more and more years passed, I became more determined to figure out how to control pain, especially without using drugs, since those just made matters worse.

It was a compulsive quest, born out of frustration. I did not expect success, yet I was finally successful, amazingly enough, and have helped others control their pain, too. That happy ending gave a worthwhile purpose to my years of suffering.

My chronic pain began in elementary school, back in the 1960s. I had an autoimmune disease that was slowly destroying my parotid glands. The parotids are the large salivary glands located in front of the ears, along the jaw line. From elementary school on, my glands cycled between periods of calm to inflammation and infection.

The trigeminal nerves (right and left), which are said to produce more pain than any other nerves in the body, process feelings for the head and face, the teeth (think how painful a toothache can be), and the cornea of the eyes (decidedly the most densely packed area of pain neurons on our body). Feelings from the parotid glands are also served by the trigeminal nerves. From personal experience, only the spinal cord itself can create more pain than the trigeminal nerve.

The autoimmune condition of my parotid glands worsened over time, and my trigeminal nerves (both sides of the face) made sure I knew it. Producing saliva was painful because it became trapped inside the glands, which were riddled with holes. Saliva would build up inside with no way to exit, causing the glands to swell to the point of tearing (major stimulation for the trigeminal nerves). The swelling was so great that the glands and escaping fluid pushed out into my face and down my neck. The swelling even pushed outward against my external ears, pushing them away from my skull. My ears felt like they were being torn away. Just thinking about eating or drinking, or actually doing either, was unbearable due to the instant saliva buildup, swelling, pushing and tearing.

While on narcotic painkillers for the trigeminal nerve pain back in the mid 1970's, I realized that although the meds dulled my senses, I still felt pain through the narcotic fog. Being essentially semi-unconscious, I could not moan and groan, yet I still experienced pain.

I was on the highest dose possible, yet it just wasn't helping. Eventually, I stopped taking the pills despite the pain. As it turned out, freeing my body of narcotics that week unwittingly set the stage for my first, although brief encounter with mindfulness techniques for stopping chronic pain.

It was 1977, and I was literally dying from the worst parotid/trigeminal nerve flare up, which continued for 13 days and nights without a moment's break. My constant severe pain, and the inability to open my mouth due to the swelling, prevented me from eating more than a few spoonfuls of mashed potato per day. Even the process of drinking water through a straw was difficult because water triggered salivation, intensifying my extreme pain. I was 5'7", and due to lack of food, I kept losing weight until I was down to only 83 pounds at my last doctor's visit. My reflection in the mirror showed skin covering only bones. I kept losing weight.

The intense pain was beyond all consuming. Words cannot express it. Pain had taken on the quality of musical notes for me. I sensed deep-pitched sounding pain and very high-pitched sounding pain, just as a piano has low and high notes, plus I sensed all the notes in between. This went on day and night, non-stop.

One afternoon, I believed that any pain had to be better than this, even if it were only imaginary. I imagined with all the focus I could muster, while lying on my back in bed, that something was twisting my right arm off. I forced myself to believe it. I gave every bit of my attention to the task of visualizing how it might look and feel, both physically and emotionally. I imagined with total concentration that the twisting was 'real'. Then I imagined that the arm was off. I imagined the pain that my shoulder might feel. I imagined what it looked like. I felt its imaginary searing pain, as if it were actually real. I kept intensely focusing and focusing....

Suddenly, what I never expected to happen happened. The inhumane pain from my parotid gland's trigeminal nerve neurons, which had been driving me insane all of those days and nights, actually stopped! Nothing hurt!

16

I became aware of an emotional high that filled every cell of my body. I experienced waves of comfort coursing throughout the full length of my body. Comfort extended from my head to my toes, and out to my fingertips. I experienced a rush of peace and inner joy. Most importantly, pain had stopped! Yes, it had stopped! For a moment.

Unfortunately, freedom from pain lasted for only a few moments, but its absence was stark, and I have remembered it throughout my lifetime as if it were yesterday. As I lie there, enduring the trigeminal nerve pain yet again, I took some comfort in the realization that at least I stopped pain somehow, for however briefly. I had new hope!

Before that short break from the pain, I had given up completely. Following those few moments of success, and armed with this new hope, I wanted to live. I decided to take the risk and let the doctor experiment with whatever surgical procedures he could try in order to end the pain. Luckily, he came up with an experiment that worked well for both of my parotid glands. I continued to lose weight, so we thought we had waited too long to operate, yet eventually I regained weight, and recovered.

Due to the intense suffering for two weeks due to my painful parotid glands in 1977, I discovered that using highly intentioned thought somehow made it possible to stop pain. Visualization is one key for unlocking our internal, intrinsic power against pain.

I hoped to perfect it, so I could stop pain for an extended period of time, instead of only a few moments. Although decades followed with many more episodes of serious pain, including five weeks of spinal cord pain, plus many surgeries, it was difficult to recreate the right conditions for visually controlling pain.

Continuing with trial and error, I noticed that imaging how nice it would feel to be healed and pain-free 'six weeks from now' brought temporary pain relief. That was a start in the right direction, and it worked for many different causes and types of relatively minor pain. Yet chronic pain continued to control me more and more. I eventually developed hypersensitivity to pain, which continued for a couple of decades.

The trigger for success in my quest for pain control unwittingly began when I injured my right foot in 2004. All of the ligaments that held four of my toes to that foot were torn completely. Pain renewed itself every time I stepped onto that foot, or when bed sheets, socks, or shoes touched it, or when something bent the toes.

Pain was intense day and night. Even when I rested my foot, the pain continued. I effectively had a chronic condition with recurring and lingering acute pain that did not know how to stop; a chronic condition which created both recurring acute and chronic pain.

The ligaments remained torn, and the bones didn't know where to fit, or how to stay there. I was told I shouldn't walk barefooted ever again, and that my foot would remain painful for life. No visualizations, distractions, or sending surges of joy and peace through my body could end the pain for any effective period of time. The doctor said the ligaments could not be fixed, but that wearing an air cast boot for a while might help.

The rocker bottom of the air cast boot helped keep my toes from bending, held all of the bones comfortably in place, and made walking more comfortable. Following air cast therapy, I wore shoes with rocker bottoms nearly every minute of every day, except while sleeping or standing in the shower.

To hold the bed covers high above my feet, I experimented with odds and ends, finally constructing a frame that fit across the foot of my bed to drape the covers over, so I could finally sleep through the night.

Suffering from my foot injury's relentless chronic pain for six years inadvertently triggered my discovering all the intrinsic techniques we are born with, both mentally and physically, for controlling our own chronic pain.

My slow-motion quantum leap in pain control finally came in 2010, once I noticed that sometimes it didn't hurt to stand in the shower, or later to briefly walk barefooted across the tiled bathroom floor.

I hadn't been able to walk barefooted without pain, yet suddenly, now there were times that I could, and those times were becoming more frequent. Eventually, I could even walk in regular, flat street shoes for a few hours at a time before feeling pain. My reality changed.

After six years of pain, to suddenly not feel pain in my foot was unbelievable. I tried to figure out what had changed. I had no clue. The ligaments had not healed. Even though it had been years, the joints were still swollen from inflammation. I was determined to figure out what was making pain control possible, to perfect it, and keep the pain away indefinitely, not just hours.

While I alternated between wearing rocker bottom and flat street shoes, I tried to remain alert enough to notice what aspect of my condition had changed. After a few months, my answer finally came.

After running errands in street shoes and returning home in pain, as usual, this time I noticed that when I sat down, I automatically touched the top of my shoe, directly above the painful area, with my hand. When my hand touched the shoe, the pain stopped instantly.

I couldn't believe it. The moment I lightly touched my shoe/foot, the pain stopped. How could that be? It didn't make logical sense (based on my definition of reality at the time), so it had to be coincidental.

Was this similar to when a mother softly kisses her young child's scratched knee to make it better - and the child believes it is all better? Did the child accept his scratch felt better only because his mom told him it would, or did the soft kiss actually make the pain stop?

Controlling pain ran against my instinctive sense of reality. Even though every single time I lightly touched my foot, pain relief was reproducibly and predictably immediate, my instincts set up a wall of denial. I still believed that pain's control over me was absolute.

Instincts fought so hard to prevent a split in my mind's reality that it took two more years for me to become thoroughly convinced that my control over pain was actually *real*.

Also in 2010, while pain control was slowly emerging in the background of my mind, people were visiting my home to contemplate mindfulness, spirituality, and spend an hour or two reducing stress. Through word of mouth, others came to see me for advice about recovering from posttraumatic stress disorder (PTSD), since I had personally recovered from PTSD fifteen years earlier.

By December 2010, I became aware that a large percentage of inmates at our local jail were there on drug charges. I wondered if their drug use was due to self-medication for relieving their suffering from PTSD. I hoped I could help. (Before I understood pain control.)

I called the local jail to ask for permission to give a talk about PTSD recovery. I hoped they would say yes, yet at the same time I hoped they would say no because jails seemed like scary places. They invited me to come for an interview in January. Once there, it was scary, yet something about it felt right. I was unwittingly stepping into a second branch of my life's primary purpose.

I needed to have an actual business in order to give my talk, so my company, Creating Balance Institute, got its start. Presuming the inmates' drug use could be related to PTSD, I gave a talk of hope, letting them know that, if it applied to any of them, they could recover from PTSD (as I had done), even if they have been told they can't (as I had been). I let them know they could find comfort and inner peace again without needing to self-medicate with drugs that might lead to addiction, which rather than helping, as they know, only compounds the seriousness of their situation.

One short talk that afternoon in January 2011 expanded into my teaching as a volunteer at the jail until Thanksgiving that November. Based on my work with the inmates, I developed twelve different educational, science-based classes for mindfulness-based stress recovery, including a class for recovery from PTSD. 2011 became the most meaningful year of my entire life, bar none.

I continued developing the classes and taught them at a local theater for a three-month series ending in May 2012. Once the last class of that series was completed, I told my students that I planned to develop a thirteenth class to teach pain control. We wondered if I taught my chronic pain control techniques to others, would they be able to control their pain, too? One of my students at the theater wondered if the techniques could help burn victims, and I wondered if having the skills would help surgery recovery pain. There were many questions.

Since these pain control techniques were still mysterious to me in 2012, and I was just beginning to believe the effects were actually real, I told them I needed time for more research and development before my pain control class could be ready. I certainly didn't imagine that this book would be a result.

Two significant breakthroughs that would solidify pain control happened back-to-back in July 2012. I was stung by a wasp on my shoulder blade, and later I seriously injured my left knee. Even though the causes and their types of pain were very different, I stopped their pain within minutes. Further, the knee injury was severe enough that I would get my answer about pain control's effectiveness for a very serious surgery recovery by that December.

Starting with the wasp sting, a contractor friend and I were working together on a project in my backyard, when the wasp stung me on the shoulder blade. My friend identified it as a wasp when he flicked it off of my shirt. I considered this stinging pain on my back to be yet another opportunity for testing my chronic pain control skills.

Since I couldn't touch it, I wanted to see if I could do something 'mentally' to stop the stinging. Everybody knows you can't stop a wasp sting by just thinking about it, and I knew that, too. Yet I was on a mission and didn't want to presume I already knew; by July 2012, I was fairly practiced at questioning and overriding any instincts about the permanence of pain. My contractor friend watched as I closed my eyes, took a conscious breath, and sent joy and pleasure coursing through my body, reminiscent of my experience in 1977.

I was blown away when the stinging stopped after only a few moments, seconds really. I started laughing, as I told my friend it had actually worked! Oops - the stinging instantly came back.

I assumed it came back because I had broken my concentration. We were still laughing while I tried again. The stinging stopped again. I kept focusing on creating the surge of joy throughout my body, plus other mindfulness-based techniques I had developed over the years, for about 90 seconds before I stopped concentrating. That time the pain didn't return, ever! We couldn't believe it. I 'mentally' stopped pain. I had finally accomplished my 1977 goal of being able to think or visualize away pain for an extended period of time, not just moments.

A week or two later, while we were still working on the project in my backyard, my feet became entangled in a plastic loop that was lying on the ground. They became so entangled that I stumbled, struggled to regain my balance, and fell as I felt my left knee rip apart inside. That rip radiated throughout my whole body.

While walking, I no longer knew where my left foot was going to land. Instead of a cheery swagger to my step, I had a tipsy stagger to my step. Yet I controlled the pain really well with the touching and mindfulness techniques I had been developing. Pain was not an issue at all. I realized that was strange, but I was happy with it. I was trusting my skills more, and I felt more convinced that they were real and not just coincidental.

I told one of my doctors about my new skills. I was visiting her for a relatively minor medical procedure. To test my skills, she agreed to not give me the local anesthetic shot. I used my mind in the same way I did with the wasp sting, and I didn't feel pain from the little incision she had to make. Because that procedure didn't hurt, she wondered if there might be something wrong with me, like perhaps I had a form of neuropathy.

That minor procedure should have hurt. Was there something wrong with my nervous system?

Since my gait was so unstable, something in my knee was probably torn, so I went to see a knee doctor. I thought he'd suggest physical therapy to strengthen the knee, but I needed total joint replacement surgery.

Hearing the word 'surgery' sent a shiver down my spine, perhaps due to apprehension. I also remembered back to that evening in May, at the theater, when I mentioned wondering if my techniques could help serious surgery recovery pain. Big mistake. The Universe was listening, and it responded. Want it or not, I was going to find out.

Since my techniques had taken care of foot pain, a wasp sting, mangled knee pain, and a minor medical procedure, maybe it could work for surgery recovery pain, too. I told my knee doctor I was excited to use this knee surgery to test my narcotic-free pain control skills.

He said this particular surgery was probably the most painful type of knee surgery I could have. He and his assistant were certain I would need narcotics during recovery to control the pain. I let them know I was determined not to use any narcotics and was glad it was a surgery that would really test my skills. I hoped my enthusiasm for doing this would replace my fear of the surgery. Plus, I hoped these techniques would develop into the best ways for preventing narcotic or opioid abuse. We scheduled the surgery.

As if knee surgery recovery alone weren't enough for my personal pain control research and development, about three weeks before the surgery date, I lifted a thin, yet relatively heavy, 42-pound carton containing an unassembled, wooden tea cart. The box slipped out of my hands, and its full weight descended vertically onto the top of my bare, left foot. It bounced and crashed onto my foot again, before falling over, onto the floor. My left foot was in so much pain.

I was afraid the box had broken my foot in those two places. How could I recover from the left knee replacement surgery if I had a broken left foot? I was frantic and extremely concerned that my doctor would have to cancel my surgery. I sat down to check for any obviously broken bones. There didn't seem to be any, even though the pain was that intense.

I remembered how stress intensifies pain. I observed how high my stress and anger levels were. I calmed down immediately. Then I remembered to try my new touching technique. Within a minute or two of touching, the pain from the top of my left foot completely stopped, literally. It felt as if nothing at all had happened to it. I couldn't believe it! Just how effective was this?

I had a pair of winter street shoes with a high profile. I thought that if I were to pull those shoes on, the high, snug top would fit very tightly across these two new injuries. I shuttered to think how painful stuffing my newly injured foot into one of those tight shoes might be, yet I couldn't resist the challenge. My purpose remained to test the techniques for my students' benefit. (Thinking of a positive reason for feeling pain helps reduce pain.)

Would touching stop the pain enough for me to pull on the tight, high-topped shoes? Could I then control the pain well enough to walk around in them?

I tried to pull the left shoe on. Yes! I easily pulled the shoe on over the injuries. My foot didn't hurt. And I could walk around without feeling any pain. Ridiculous.

That seemed so bizarre! Pain control kept blowing my mind. It was thrilling, too, because I finally knew for absolute certainty that I had significant control over pain. My foot turned nearly black from the bruising, but its pain did not return. There would be zero reason to postpone surgery.

Actually, because pain now seemed easy to control, my apprehension about the knee surgery, or for future surgeries in general, subsided. It had taken me 35 years since 1977 before I could finally control pain with my mind, and amazingly enough, a touch.

Until recently, recovering from PTSD seemed unrelated to pain control, but recovery from intense, long-term stress is related to recovery from chronic pain and drug abuse.

My emotional and physical suffering since the 1960's had a true purpose. Whenever anything seems only negative, hindsight or giving it enough time may reveal surprisingly positive net gains. Sometimes suffering presents the gifts of strength and understanding that can be gained no other way.

Immersion in developing and teaching stress reduction classes at the jail and theater, with pain control methods developing simultaneously and mysteriously in the background on their own, appeared to be linked. While I was not aware of it at the time, each contributed to the success of the other. Stumbling over and tripping when I blew out my knee also rammed me face-first into that invisible link between stress and pain, while I kept moving smoothly on my journey for decades, as if it were somehow planned all along.

So far, it had been a long journey of blindly searching for a solution that might not have even been there. Yet techniques for pain control without using narcotics, and effective solutions for PTSD recovery without self-medicating truly were there to be discovered. The journey proved extraordinarily worthwhile, for me and for many others.

The Joy of Surgery Recovery

The day for left knee replacement finally came and my doctor gave me permission to walk as soon as I woke up from the anesthesia. The surgery was a great success and in my hospital room, the moment finally came for me to wake up, be brave, and test my pain control skills on my new knee.

Technically, I was required to have one nurse on each side, supporting me so I wouldn't fall, making certain the new knee joint was stable before taking my first steps. However, the nurses did not want me to get out of bed so soon. They thought I should wait until the next day. I told them that my doctor had given me permission to get up right away.

They felt very uneasy, and moved to the far corner of my room to discuss it privately, wondering if they should give in.

One of them said, "Maybe she needs to use the restroom."

The room wasn't very big. I heard that.

"Yes, yes! I have to use the restroom!"

Laughing, yet still concerned, they came over. Each took an arm to help me rise up and onto my legs. My knees were so stable. I took a step with my left foot, applying full weight onto my new Titanium knee, and WOW! There was No Pain! Walking felt great. The joy coursing through my body was truly exhilarating!

Even though I wanted them to, one of the doctors wouldn't allow the nurses to remove the IV narcotic drip from surgery. On the phone, I begged the doctor to let them remove the line, but he would only allow them to reduce the flow. They lowered it so there was just enough flowing through the line to keep it from clogging. The doctor said that it was not enough of a flow to give me an effective dose, so it was the same thing as not using narcotics. He said I had to keep it in until the next day. So, being crafty, at one minute past midnight that night (technically the 'next' day), the nurses removed the line to help me become truly narcotic-free as soon as possible.

My knee surgeon, anesthesiologist, the hospital nurses on my floor, my physical therapists (except for one), and I were amazed and thrilled by how fast my recovery was progressing. The nurses on my floor nicknamed me Super Star, as I power walked up and down the hallways, sometimes fake-racing with the nurses for fun.

My doctor told me that he and my anesthesiologist watched me walking the halls, saying that, even though they knew which knee they operated on, they could not tell it by my gait. They could not detect a limp, which said a lot. I loved my essentially painless recovery. I didn't need pain meds or even acetaminophen during the whole recovery process.

My recovery went really well. My physical therapists were impressed. If a physical therapy exercise hurt, we paused while I applied my touch, and continued without pain. It was fun. Recovery was fast. It was a joy.

At my follow-up office visit in 2013, my knee doctor seemed to want proof. Jokingly, he asked if I could walk across the (minimally carpeted) floor on my knees. Of course, I wouldn't be able to, he must have been thinking. I figured, why assume? I got down on my knees and without using my hands, walked around on the floor. It didn't hurt! We were both amazed and it was profound.

He said that if anyone could prove pain really could be controlled, that was me, and he wondered if I could teach my techniques to others, so they could relieve their surgery recovery pain, too. We didn't know if teaching it would be effective at all, but we agreed that if teaching it were effective, and the techniques ended up helping at least 40% of students, then it would be a success.

Feeling urgency to help others suffering from chronic pain and wondering if I actually could help anyone by teaching it, I developed a workshop which included instructions for how to touch away pain, plus basic mindfulness techniques.

To offer this to people suffering from chronic pain, I rented a small office and advertised locally on Craigslist, asking volunteers for their cooperation to test these techniques on their pain. They suffered from diabetic neuropathy, fibromyalgia, spinal nerve pain (with and without implanted, electrical nerve stimulators), or serious bone deformity. We discovered they could successfully relieve their own pain by correctly touching the areas that hurt. Yes, if I taught it to them, they could learn how to control their pain and fairly quickly.

This pain control part of my business became a real passion. I needed to give it a name. I realized there was an underlying theme in all that I taught. There was a common, yet nearly invisible thread that ties all of my educational, stress reduction and pain control classes together. It was the fact that we learn to live life more lusciously by controlling long-term stress from within us. All the answers and all the tools we need for creating balance already exist 'within' us. 'Within' is the Key. It means that if the answers and tools are within, they are a part of our nature, they are 'intrinsic'.

Since the tools are within us, controlling long-term stress is 'intrinsic'; it is a natural part of us. This applies to most types of suffering, both emotional and physical. That chronic pain control is also accomplished entirely from within reinforces the significance of the underlying, fundamental, 'intrinsic' theme for not only the techniques I teach, but for how we experience everything in life. Creating Balance Is Intrinsic for Us All.

We only need to learn how to access and use those tools. Education for learning how to direct change is essential. I named the therapeutically educational branch of my CBi business for stress recovery and chronic pain control, CB Intrinsic (also CBi). Hence, my pain control methods became the CB Intrinsic Touch and Mindfulness-based Pain Control techniques.

Eventually, I rented booths at holistic or alternative medicine expos, asking about a dozen passers-by if they were in pain. I was surprised by how many people suffer from painful knees, shoulders, necks, hips and lower backs. To help them with their chronic pain, I asked their permission to test the CBi Touch (or the Touch) where they hurt, and every person I asked agreed to let me try.

Amazingly, the Touch worked for all but one of them, and it worked within minutes. These people were not using pain medications and just dealt with either chronic pain or relentless discomfort. As I applied the Touch, and taught them how to do it for themselves, their pain diminished or disappeared. I was so excited as their frowns turned to smiles.

For the people that periodically answered my Craigslist ads, and to the passers-by at the expos, I only volunteered the CBi Touch. Its quick application was enough to ease their discomfort, and perhaps put hope back in their lives. It would have taken too many hours to teach the mindfulness-based techniques.

In the fall of 2013, I rented and furnished a classroom for teaching all of my CB Intrinsic therapeutic, stress recovery classes. I was surprised that over 90% of my students for stress recovery also suffered from chronic pain. Before starting each course, I first taught students how to apply the CBi Touch, so they could be more comfortable during the classes. It worked extraordinarily well for almost all of my students suffering from chronic pain. So yes, these skills were 'skills' that others could learn, and it was far more successful than my knee doctor and I had hoped it could be.

It is difficult to believe that relief may be just a Touch away. I could walk barefooted as much as I wanted, and I didn't need to wear my rocker bottom shoes anymore.

The Touch was so effective that by the end of 2014, I removed the cover-lift frame from the foot of my bed. At that time, I only knew that these techniques could stop pain. In 2015, one of my pain control students suggested I write a book describing all of the CBi pain control techniques to be able to reach more people. I didn't know how to write a book, but I tried and finished it in 2016.

After reading my first book, someone suggested I back up my techniques with science. I began studying the literature in neuroscience journals and discovered my techniques are in line with current research findings. There was so much relatively recent neuroscience research in the journals that supports how the Touch works, I collected hundreds of articles. I continued searching in cognitive neuroscience research journals to find supporting research for the mindfulness techniques, too.

As I continued teaching my stress reduction courses and the Touch, reading and collecting more research articles to learn more of the neurobiology behind my pain control techniques, coincidences began happening again.

In February 2017, I discovered the CBi Touch can also promote healing for weakened muscles. As the months passed, more coincidences brought out evidence showing that this was indeed the case. I began writing my second chronic pain control book in the fall of 2017.

Stopping pain is not a 'cure', yet depending on the condition and an individual's circumstances, regaining muscle or gland function, i.e., a gain-in-function, can accompany intrinsic pain control techniques.
Gain-In-Function Is Huge.

Gain-In-Function Connection

I personally experienced the pain/muscle connection when, beginning in April 2015 and recurring for nearly two years, my lower back kept going out. The pain included pinched spinal nerve and cauda equina pain, so it could reach very intense levels. Each of three or four episodes lasted a few weeks, and they resolved on their own by using the Touch.

In November 2016, my back went out again, yet it was much more serious that time. While sitting on the couch and trying to stand up, it suddenly felt as if both of my legs had fused into one. I felt like a mermaid must feel. I could only hobble, and it was difficult to move my legs apart to walk. My muscles weren't working.

Dealing with pain is one thing, while the consequences from losing function (how well muscles work) and not being able to walk is orders of magnitude or is extremely worse than just experiencing pain. This was very serious. I decided to not apply the Touch, so the acute pain could help me know whether or not things were getting better, and to help me describe the condition to a doctor.

It was not possible to take normal walking strides. Along their length, my legs sort of felt glued to each other. I could only shuffle, bending my ankles and feet to take tiny steps. I believe I wasn't too fearful because I viewed anything related to chronic pain conditions as instructive, and whatever I experienced I viewed as potentially helpful for my students. A genuinely positive attitude helps reduce pain.

After a few days, the mermaid feeling left, yet my legs worked like scissors with adhesive stuck between the blades. It was really hard to separate them to walk, or to get dressed, lean over, go up or down stairs, stand up from a sitting position, etc.

The pain was periodically very intense, concentrated mostly at my lower back, both hips, and my left leg. My left tibia and fibula, plus the upper half of the femur at times felt like they were red hot fireplace pokers. The pain was strong, and it took a lot of skill to not let it overwhelm me.

I finally met with one doctor, who referred me to the next and the next, until we covered all the bases, and I had a full diagnosis. We figured out the best options for back surgery. Finally, by the end of January 2017, all that was left to do was schedule the surgery.

With the diagnoses completed, and while my three fireplace poker bones were burning red hot, I applied the Touch to my lower back and both hips. I leaned over as much as I could to apply it to my left thigh. I could bend over only enough for my fingertips to reach the top part of my left knee. I applied the Touch to the front, back, and all around my left thigh a well as I could. I was not surprised that the pain stopped immediately. I hoped the relief would last at least a week or two.

I procrastinated scheduling the surgery because, even though I needed it, I was afraid of back surgery. Three or four days passed while the most amazing and unexpected thing was happening. My legs began working really well, and I could bend at the waist. My hips bent so well that I could easily touch the floor. Instead of only shuffling, my legs could walk. It was unbelievable. Yet again.

I called the doctor's office, early the first week of February 2017, and told the receptionist that I had applied the Touch a few days earlier, thinking it might give me relief from the pain for a couple of weeks before surgery. I also told her that I couldn't believe it, but in addition to no pain, I was regaining muscle function. I told her that even though I thought the symptoms would all return in a week or two, I didn't want to schedule the surgery just yet. I wanted to wait and see.

She said that sometimes patients spontaneously recover. She said they didn't know why, but that it was okay to wait a little while before scheduling back surgery.

Actually, full function returned. Applying the Touch initiated that rapid recovery. The pain stopped instantly, as I expected, but improved muscle function surprised me. Later, my chiropractor mentioned that they know pain restricts muscle function, so it made sense to him that removing pain might help me regain function.

I struggled with not understanding why my system reset itself so completely after only applying the Touch. It was too hard to believe the incredible changes. No pain and my legs worked again, after suffering pain for a couple of months with my muscles not working right? It was too much for me to process. My legs had been stuck together, and I couldn't even lean over. As it turns out, regaining muscle function was actually not so strange.

About four months later, NBC Nightly News featured surprising research results from Dr. Kim Bullock, a Stanford Neuropsychiatrist. Dr. Bullock studies reducing patients' anxiety symptoms, and strengthening weakened muscles using virtual reality (VR) treatments. Concurrent with VR treatments for anxiety and muscle strengthening treatments, patients were experiencing a reduction in chronic pain, lasting from weeks to months. Dr. Bullock was surprised to find the connection between lowering anxiety (stress), gaining muscle function, and relieving chronic pain. (See Author's Notes, p. 233.)

I was amazed that the surprising link between controlling pain and regaining muscle function, which I experienced firsthand, was also noticed by a Stanford Neuropsychiatrist through her patients. Even more validation of muscle/gland gain-in-function followed.

A couple of months after learning about Dr. Bullock's results, someone suffering from painful cystic fibrosis (CF) symptoms asked for my help. The Touch stopped the pain, as expected, and it also helped improve many other symptoms from CF complications.

Over a few months, it became apparent that the CF pain had been contributing to secondary conditions related to partial loss of intestinal muscle and gland function. Controlling the pain allowed regaining significant muscle and gland function, along with other improvements, such as being able to sleep better and live life more lusciously. Improvements continued for my CF student.

Instead of pain relief lasting only a couple of weeks, CBi techniques kept pain away and function normal, for over three years. MRI showed the condition was very severe, even though pain and function were not an issue.

Lowering stress levels, diminishing chronic pain symptoms, and helping reduce loss of muscle/gland function are consistently and positively correlated.

The CBi Touch is effective all by itself, and is taught in Part II, yet as we saw when I stopped the wasp sting pain on my back, the Touch is not the only skill we can use for controlling chronic pain.

Several CB Intrinsic Mindfulness-based Pain Control (MBPC) techniques control pain by directly addressing the stress component of the pain/stress/muscle-function connection. Reducing stress has positive outcomes in most aspects of one's life. Although it's meant to be used with chronic pain control, MBPC has far-reaching, positive impacts on quality of life, too.

The ten CBi mindfulness techniques take time to explain, yet they are all simple to use and easily become second nature. Chronic pain loses out because mindfulness-based pain control techniques can *restore* the nervous system's normal ability to stop pain. The CBi Touch, along with MBPC techniques positively impact every component necessary for helping the nervous system normalize the way it processes pain again, plus they may improve weakened muscle or gland function.

Let's consider some ways that the nervous system routinely controls pain and apply that to better understand how the Touch and MBPC might work.

How the CBi Touch Works

Since I studied Neurobiology to earn my Masters' degree back in 2001, I realized that something about the Touch might be mentioned in my old textbooks that are still sitting on my shelf. I checked and found clues.

The Gate Control Theory of Pain was a hypothesis proposed by MIT professors Patrick David Wall (neuroscientist) and Ronald Melzack (psychologist) positing that a light touch could modify pain. In 1965, their paper was published in the prestigious scientific journal Science.[1] Based on the principles of their Gate Control Theory of pain, Dr. Wall went on to develop TENS or the Transcutaneous Electrical Nerve Stimulator, which some doctors use to help patients alleviate their pain.

Related to the light touch, our graduate studies in 2000 covered the process for controlling pain by rubbing a hurt area. We studied the Wide Dynamic Range (WDR) neurons found in the spinal cord and examined the role they play in sending signals from touch, temperature and pain neurons up toward the brain for processing. But they can send only one of those types of signals at a time.

When we immediately rub a painful, bumped elbow or stubbed toe, the WDRs can only receive nerve signals about the pain or about the rubbing. The decision is

---

[1] Melzack, R, Wall, PD. 1965. Pain mechanisms: a new theory. *Science.* 150(3699):971 979

made in the spinal cord whether the WDRs will send signals about rubbing to the brain, instead of pain from the stubbed or bumped pain. Once the WDRs send rub signals to the brain, our awareness of pain is at the least reduced, if some of the pain signals still get through, or it is stopped completely.

Yet the response at the spinal cord to a rubbing touch is different from the response to light touch because rubbing is only effective with bumps and stubs. Rubbing stimulates a different set of neurons than a light touch will stimulate.

We know through experience that stimulating rubbing neurons has not been effective against chronic pain. Many people use deep pressure rubs where their chronic pain hurts, rubbing in equal measure to the pain. It gives emotional relief. But no matter how hard we rub an area with chronic pain, the pain does not stop. Only touching lightly works with chronic pain.

What happens at the spinal cord to determine which signals the WDRs send up toward the brain? We need more background to try to understand.

Neurons are the primary cells of the nervous system. Pain sensing neurons that react to painful stimulus are called 'nociceptors'. Processing pain signals eventually leads to the sensation of pain in the brain.[2] Nociceptors are located in skin, muscle, bone, joints and organs, but interestingly, not in the brain. Nociceptors are responsible for initiating pain signals that are sent the

[2] Dubin, AE, Patapoutain, A. Nociceptors: the sensors of the pain pathway. 2010. *J Clin Invest.* 120(11):3760-3772. doi: 10.1172/JCI42843

full distance of that pain neuron inside its nerve to the spinal cord. (Trigeminal neurons for the face and head send pain and touch signals to the brainstem, instead of the spinal cord - beyond this book's scope.)

The neurons we stimulate for the CB Intrinsic Touch also begin in the skin and span all the way to the spinal cord, within the same nerves as the nociceptors (pain neurons). Once activated by faint vibrations on the skin, those light touch neurons eventually interact with neighboring neurons at the spinal cord.

They interact with the pain neurons to inhibit or turn off pain signals arriving at the cord at the same time. Perhaps to make certain pain is turned off, they stimulate little neurons inside the cord, called interneurons, that also inhibit signals from those same pain neurons. Pain signals are effectively turned off by that double punch of inhibition, preventing their signals from reaching the WDR neurons. Signals for the light touch win the competition and rise up in the WDRs toward the brain. We feel the tickle of the light touch vibrations, not pain.

When we stub a toe and rub it, a similar process takes place at the cord when the rub signals out compete pain signals. We perceive the rub, but not the pain.

The fact that the WDRs are restricted to carrying only one type of signal at a time (touch, temp or pain) toward the brain also helps ensure we have less chance of feeling pain when there is competition from a rub or light touch.

The nervous system gives signals from a light touch priority over signals from chronic pain, perhaps in the same way it prefers signals from the strong pressure of a rubbed elbow over the pain of a bumped elbow. We can train our nervous system to consistently prioritize light touch neurons over chronic pain neurons.

How this works is much more complicated than I presented here. Furry animals are used in research to learn the facts about light touch neurons. (The Touch works on our furry pets' pain, too. (See Furry Pets' Pain, p. 80.) Animals do not display the placebo effect. Since interactions of the Touch with pain neurons happen at the spinal cord, the brain is not involved in making the Touch work, so the Touch is technically not impacted by placebo effect in humans either. Thinking, understanding, and/or believing in the Touch are not necessary for it to work.

The power residing within a simple, slowly applied light touch is impressive, and it's still hard for me to believe, every single time I use it. Try the Touch on your furry pet's pain. Pets might not like the tickle initially, but gently persist. Eventually your pet may connect loss of pain with your Touch and come to you voluntarily for help. My cat finally figured it out and found tremendous relief from his arthritic pain.

It's curious how we doubt that the light touch can work, but we easily believe and do not doubt that rubbing with strong pressure should work for chronic pain, even though it doesn't. It may go against the grain, but we actually can believe in the Touch. And thinking back, I didn't remember learning about the Gate Control Theory of Pain in graduate school, yet there it was in my textbooks. Applying it now means I luckily don't suffer from some strange neuropathy that allowed only me to control pain, as one of my doctors and I feared.

For diminishing chronic pain, the light touch neurons found in the skin compete successfully against pain neurons for selection by the WDRs of the spinal cord. They win the competition often enough that we can use them at will to control chronic pain. We feel sensations from the light touch rather than pain because those touch neurons have taken direct and indirect actions to inhibit or prevent pain neurons from communicating with the WDRs.

When we have an itch, we rapidly scratch it to make the itch stop. When it itches later, we scratch it again. Rapid scratching is a type of touch. The scratch is felt, while the itch is forgotten. From the perspective of the brain, pain and itch are similar. Perhaps it makes sense that in the same way scratching controls an itch, another type of touch is meant to control pain. But scratching is instinctive, and using the Touch isn't.

Culturally, we are conditioned to believe we are at pain's mercy. But the fact is there are intrinsic ways for lessening, relieving, and even stopping chronic pain. It's difficult to believe because it is the opposite of what we experience. That we are at the mercy of pain, that we need a pill or an outside action, and that there can't be an intrinsic way to stop pain are merely belief systems. Those beliefs are reinforced by what we personally experience, by pressure from our cultural beliefs, and by common sense that is based on instincts. We need to challenge those hardened beliefs. It is healthy to challenge belief systems, especially when so much is at stake. Unnecessary chronic pain and long-term stress are unhealthy.

When a little kid scrapes his knee, he and his mother often believe it will feel better once she lightly kisses it. Faint touch/no pain. We stop accepting that as we age. Believing in a light touch again or believing that a light touch stopping pain is even possible may help more people take a chance and try the Touch.

The Touch is a skill that can be developed relatively quickly. Normally, in order for pain to be felt, pain signals must travel inside nerves, from the source that initiated the painful stimulus, on up to the spinal cord. Those signals are processed and modified by neurons within the spinal cord. For further processing, the modified information continues up to reach many separate areas within the brainstem and brain. Pain is only fully perceived as 'real' after the fully processed signals reach the cortex of the brain, and thus our awareness.

Let's consider that the Touch works from the bottom-up, from the injury site up to the spinal cord. The Touch works intrinsically by preventing pain signals from traveling beyond their first interactions with the light touch and other neurons in the spinal cord. If pain signals cannot rise up to be fully processed from the spinal cord to the cortex of the brain, pain perception does not occur. That means the mind was prevented from creating that pain, so that pain never existed.

Novice students can usually learn how to perform the Touch within twenty to thirty minutes. The Bottom-Up (skin to brain) results are immediate and powerful.

CB Intrinsic MBPC techniques control pain from the top-down, which means signals from pain control centers in the brain and brainstem travel down to the spinal cord to prevent pain signals from rising up.

Incredibly, by simply changing thoughts and modifying behavior patterns, the natural, intrinsic painkilling abilities of the brain itself can significantly impede or reduce perceptions of pain, at will.

It takes many hours or days to teach MBPC basics to a novice student. Given this initially steep learning curve, reading, practicing, and repeating provides the best method for developing Top-Down MBPC skills.

During practice, MBPC techniques activate brain centers that send peace, joy, pleasure, and a new sense of well-being coursing throughout the entire body, which makes learning and mastering MBPC rewarding.

As that steep learning curve turns into a reward curve, learning and assimilating these new skills naturally become easier. Learning flows more like water running downhill, until MBPC becomes second nature. Once these techniques are mastered and that realization hits, trust in being able to wield the power of chronic pain control becomes exciting and exhilarating.

Learning and mastering MBPC skills in Part III does require a desire to do so, remembering to practice, and an open mind that allows paradigm shifting toward this healthier state of mind and new pain control mindset.

While using CB Intrinsic Touch and MBPC techniques together provides healthy options for finding relief from chronic pain, remember that sensations of pain and the condition itself are two completely different things. Merely stopping the perception of pain does not mean an injury or condition has healed or is cured.

Just as the receptionist at my neurosurgeon's office mentioned in 2017, experience teaches us that sometimes pain is somehow spontaneously silenced. How can pain be 'spontaneously' silenced? What are some fairly common ways that we know pain is being silenced? Are any of those ways understood well enough that we can apply them whenever we want to stop our chronic pain? What are our options?

CBi Pain Control Options

For a starting point, let's consider which intrinsic techniques are most effective against pain. I can explain it best by telling stories to help us imagine a few scenarios that are known to silence pain. Then we can incorporate them into our plan for controlling pain intrinsically.

Sleep takes priority over pain.

We don't feel pain during sleep. Severe pain keeps us from sleeping, but once we fall asleep, pain is not felt. If you feel pain during sleep, you are actually only dozing, and dozing doesn't stop pain.

The intensities of stress and of pain are positively correlated; high stress results in higher pain, which results in even higher stress.

Sleep is a relatively stress-free state of body and mind. Sleep is not only important for quality of life. Being able to sleep is essential for life. When someone is able to sleep, the nervous system is giving sleep a higher priority over their pain.

When pain's intensity is so great that sleep cannot be achieved, lowering stress levels, by completely releasing any tension in muscles or thoughts, is the key to finally falling asleep. Regardless, it is impractical to stay asleep 24/7 in order to control chronic pain. Although sleep is an intrinsic solution for controlling chronic pain, it isn't always practical.

'Focusing intensely' takes priority over pain.

Sleeping is not the only mental exercise we can try for controlling pain. Professional athletes may finish a goal before noticing they sustained a serious injury. With the goal accomplished, cheering begins, and the athlete mysteriously falls to the ground in pain, wondering what just happened.

In those situations, pain from an injury does not necessarily become apparent until someone's intense concentration is broken, or until their imperative goal has been completed. Does it require years of the same extensive training that professional athletes undergo before pain could be ignored in favor of the objective or goal? Or could someone block pain due to intense concentration without professional training first?

Let's consider a situation that anyone could encounter, involving intense pain and an equally intense focus on something else.

Imagine that you have a very painful knee. One beautiful spring day, you're sitting on your front porch, checking your email, and sipping iced tea. Your leg is resting on a pillowed ottoman, with your knee chilling under an ice pack.

You are distracted when you notice that a neighbor's toddler is walking around outside, all by herself. Now she is walking along the sidewalk toward your house. Once she reaches your driveway, the tulips blooming in a neighbor's yard across the street catch her eye. Instead of continuing along the sidewalk toward your house, and with her wide-eyed gaze firmly focused on the tulips, she turns to head down your driveway, presumably to cross the street on her way to the tulips.

You quickly scan the scene and consider the cars parked along both sides of your street. You also notice an oncoming car and realize the seriousness of the situation. The driver might not see this little girl as she crosses the street because the parked cars could hide her tiny frame.

In an instant, you jump up and run to grab the little girl. You call out telling her to stop, which she sort of does, but keeps walking, backwards, toward the street. It also alerts her mom to come out of their house to join you. You reach the little girl and scoop her up, struggling in your arms as the car passes. Problem solved. You were right for acting so quickly. Almost as quickly, her mother reaches you, and you place her little daughter in her arms.

That was a good deed for the day. Your heart is pounding as you take a deep breath and walk back up your driveway toward your porch, trying to clear your head to remember what you had been doing before all of that happened.

Then you remember, grimace, and silently scream to yourself, "Oh, my knee! Oh, the Pain! Oh, that was too much!"

We often forget all about pain when something else demands our fullest attention. Once the situation is over, we remember the pain. We wish we could focus that intensely again to make the pain go away.

'Imminent danger' takes priority over pain.

While hiking earlier in the day, Janice fell off of some boulders on top of a short cliff onto the rough terrain below. She was in a lot of pain and could barely walk. Her sister Mary was on the hike with her, and they both feared Janice had broken or sprained her ankle. Mary hiked around to find cell reception to notify their husbands, who planned to arrive at the camp early the next day to help Mary get Janice to the nearest hospital.

Janice was stressed and in pain to the max. It was late at night as she lay in her sleeping bag, tossing and turning, trying to sleep. The pain had been all-consuming for hours, but finally sleep overcame her and released her from the pain. About an hour later, she awoke with a start because she felt something inside the sleeping bag wiggle across her ankle. Her anxiety spiked and she froze. What was it? Had she dreamed it?

No. There it was again. It felt furry! Not good! Chipmunk? Janice scrambled out of her sleeping bag and rushed out of her tent screaming.

Hearing her cries, Mary rushed out of her tent, and found Janice trying to catch her breath, while screaming that there was something small and furry inside her sleeping bag. Still in a panic, Janice suddenly began doubling over and stumbling. Her searing, sharp, and agonizing pain returned. Janice remembered her injury.

She didn't feel the pain when she unzipped her sleeping bag and practically tore her way out of her tent. A few seconds before her realization that there might be a furry critter in her sleeping bag, and before stress and fear ramped up in her mind, the pain had already stopped. The action that stopped the pain was the relatively light touch from the critter's fur, the very instant it barely grazed her ankle. It was that faint brush with imminent danger that took priority over pain.

Focusing on getting away from the critter certainly helped stop the pain, too. All of her awareness became focused on getting away from the critter, which was seen as potential danger. The nervous system's full processing of imminent danger left no room for pain in her mind.

In this case, stress did not intensify her pain. This was imminent danger stress. That type of stress differs from long-term emotional stress. It is different from anger. Imminent danger stress commands alertness and awareness. It activates absolute focusing powers onto the present moment. There is no room for pain.

Considering these few examples helps demonstrate that according to the nervous system, pain does not always keep the highest priority. We have seen how the nervous system prioritize some types of touch over pain, and some powerful mental activities within the brain also claim priority, even over strong acute pain.

Most of us can recall times when the pain was missing. Thinking back, can you remember that while focusing intensely on something (perhaps a suspenseful scene in a movie or a critical process at work), you temporarily forgot about your pain? Did the pain actually stop, or did it continue while you were merely unaware of it? Is there a difference?

Let's use these insights into how the nervous system works to develop extraordinary skills to prudently trick the nervous system into temporarily reducing or stopping pain, and over time, hopefully heal some abnormal chronic pain processes. Tricking the nervous system is possible with understanding and know how.

Reviewing the situations in the examples, we can see that the mind takes priority away from pain during situations that are completely stress-free, essential, and imperative, or are of present and imminent danger.

Which of these offers the fastest way for stopping pain? Sleeping, focusing on goals, focusing on problem solving, or imitating imminent danger.

In Janice's case, first a light touch of fur across her ankle started the process for alerting the brain about imminent danger. At the microscopic level, the nervous system doesn't need to 'know' what caused that light touch. Neurons merely react at a biochemical level. Pain neurons were silenced by interactions with the light touch neurons and interneurons at the spinal cord level. Then stress, fear and critical thought processes instinctively took over to formulate the best strategies for avoiding the dangerous situation.

Priorities for the light touch were followed by her extraordinary alertness, awareness, clear-mindedness, and complete presence of mind, which were all-consuming and overwhelming, leaving little room for perceptions of pain, which was shut out and temporarily forgotten, until awareness levels return to normal.

Imitating imminent danger is the fastest way.

The CB Intrinsic Touch works very quickly, does not involve the brain or mind, and can have lasting results. It works from the Bottom-Up and is covered in Part II.

We cover ten CB Intrinsic Mindfulness-based Pain Control (MBCP) techniques that effectively teach the mind how to trick itself into controlling pain in Part III. Learning how is not difficult. Through neuroplasticity, MBPC leads to automatically controlling pain for months or years. It works from the Top-Down.

Part IV covers healthy partnerships in pain control. From family members to practitioners, it takes a village.

Controlling pain can have serious ramifications. We must fully understand and appreciate why taking care of each illness or condition that pain alerted us to is much more important than silencing its pain. Do not stop acute pain that still serves a purpose. Correctly distinguish between appropriate and inappropriate use of these skills. Due to the complexities involved, children and teenagers' minds are not developed fully enough to practice these skills safely or prudently. Such precautions, plus limitations are addressed in Part V.

Unlike scratching an itch to stop it, using any of these CB Intrinsic techniques to stop pain is not instinctive, but we are born with these innate abilities. We can learn how to apply these hidden abilities, while always keeping safety first. Do not apply these techniques unless or until your condition(s) is diagnosed and your doctor says it is alright to practice chronic pain control.

Let's begin with the CB Intrinsic Touch, since that is the easiest to learn, and it works relatively quickly.

Part II

CB INTRINSIC TOUCH TECHNIQUES

Intrinsic Touch Basics

The nervous system gives 'imminent danger' priority over pain.

Since pain is invisible, we cannot 'see' when these techniques work. We can only feel the void left behind as the pain reduces or stops. Therefore, to know if it is being applied correctly, it is necessary to be experiencing pain while the CB Intrinsic Touch is applied.

Whether I teach this to pain practitioners or my adult CB Intrinsic chronic pain students, I follow the same standard procedure. I apply the CBi Touch to the back of their hand and forearm. They discover how it feels on their skin. Then, they apply the Touch to the back of their hand and forearm, to imitate my application of the Touch. Once they feel confident, they test their skills on the back of my hand and forearm. That helps me know they are applying it correctly. We practice, back and forth, my application, their application, and correction until they can perform the Touch correctly. Finally, I teach them how to apply the Touch to the specific areas of their current chronic pain, on the skin or over their clothing.

Know that when the Touch is applied correctly, and the pain stops suddenly, the Touch stopped it. It was not because the pain stopped on its own. It is not a coincidence that the pain suddenly stopped while 'trying to learn' the technique. There is no need to wait for the pain to return to try again to learn the Touch. The technique worked.

Since the Touch works at the microscopic level, try thinking at the microscopic level to understand how to apply it.

By zooming in at the microscopic level, we can imagine how perspiration could cause the hands or fingers to stick to the skin. Rather than being able to glide smoothly, sticking makes the Touch rough. It works best if the hands providing the Touch are clean so they can 'glide' over the skin or clothing.

In addition, salty residue left behind from perspiration keeps moisture on the skin, which may cause the hand or skin to feel humid and warm to the touch. If there is perspiration and salty residue, both the hands and the area of skin where the Touch will be applied should be washed with soap first, using cool or cold water, and then rinsed and dried well.

The CBi Touch is NOT massage. Muscles or joints are not being rubbed or pressed. Only the tip-top surface of the skin is being slowly and very lightly touched. This is not Reiki, as the skin is physically being touched.

As with all things in nature, there are exceptions, and almost everything is expressed as a continuum or range. We are each different, so the range that works best for applying the Touch for each person may vary. Touch works optimally if it can glide lightly and smoothly, without having perspiration creating drag when we stroke slowly to activate specific painkilling neurons.

A medical doctor, who was a chronic pain control student of mine, told me that the tickle surprised him when he applied the Touch for himself. He didn't believe he could 'tickle' himself, yet just he did. We assume our beliefs are correct. We are told we can't tickle ourselves, but we can. This is new kind of touch for most people.

Next, I will give a description of how I teach the Touch to a novice student. For practitioners, this is how you might like to present the Touch to each of your patients.

I ask the student, sitting in front of me, to rest one hand on mine, palm to palm. Then I gently lower my other hand, palm-side down, until it is just barely touching the skin of his hand and forearm. I emphasize *barely touching*. (If you, the reader, would like to try this, set down the book, and without feeling the weight of your second hand, gently lower it until it *barely* touches the backside of your firsthand and/or forearm.)

Without any pressure at all, I move the fingers and palm of my hand very slowly back and forth, and all around in swirls, on the back of his hand and forearm, just barely touching. This may tickle a little bit, and he may feel a cool sensation.

The palm of my touching hand can be raised up so only the fingertips are touching and gliding, swirling in random motions along the backside of his hand and forearm (bare arm or over a shirt sleeve). I can also use the fingertips of both of my hands at the same time, swirling randomly around, along the back of my student's hand and forearm. My motions are slow, very light and relaxed. (See Pressure Range Summary, p. 75.)

By applying a bit more pressure onto the back of my student's hand and forearm, the tickling or cool sensation will stop, yet as long as contact remains very light, the Touch is still being applied correctly at this end of the effective Touch range. I move my hand and fingers in circles or any combination of movements.

I would not call this a 'reassuring' type of touch because reassuring implies too much pressure would be applied. Barely a fraction of the weight of my hand is ever applied – we could say there is no 'weight' to the Touch, even with a slight increase in pressure. It needs to remain practically weightless to stay within the 'imminent danger' zone necessary for stopping chronic pain.

I check to see if the student can imitate my actions. He practices the same techniques on the back of his hand and forearm, trying to make it feel the same as it did when I applied the Touch for him. Once he is ready, he practices the Touch on the back of my hand and forearm. I give feedback while we use trial and error.

When first applying the Touch, some students come to me with a 'heavy' hand. Construction workers apply more pressure than we need, partly because they are accustomed to applying great force with their hands. They lift and operate heavy equipment and tools. They apply great force all day long. Their muscles may have compromised fine, delicate touch in exchange for firmness and strength. They are not accustomed to touching something as lightly as this, but success is just a matter of becoming more familiar with it.

As it is with everything else, what constitutes 'light' for each person is subjective; it depends on and is relative to their own abilities and experience. Performing the CBi Touch skills correctly takes practice and patience, so we try again and again until his touch is not only relatively light to his experience and ability, but empirically, measurably 'light'.

If his touch remains heavy, we will practice applying the Touch weightlessly to the tops of the hairs on his arm, without touching the skin below. Next, he will lightly touch the skin below, and progress until he believes he can apply a truly weightless touch. We test it to see if he can apply the Touch correctly to the back of my hand and forearm. He will practice the Touch on his own hand and forearm, and then on mine, until he can create the same tickle and sometimes cool sensation that are hallmarks of the lightest CBi Touch techniques.

If this process takes much longer than 15 minutes, we take a break for a few minutes because the skin might become temporarily fatigued or insensitive to the Touch. We give the skin time to reset.

Touch Basics for the Reader

I cannot test the heaviness of the reader's hand. Let's assume you have a heavy hand or a heavy touch, and we'll begin with a visualization.

Imagine how lightly your fingers would have to touch the skin of a beating drum to feel its vibrations without dampening the sound. If you pressed any harder, you would feel the leather itself, but that would dampen the sound.

Imagine at the microscopic level, as your skin barely touches the beating drum skin, whose vibrating leather rises up against the surface of your fingers, and falls, rises and falls. Applying no weight to your fingers, you sense only the peak of these vibrations. Dampening the drum's sound to any degree would let you know you are touching it with too much pressure. Imitating that very lightest touch on the drum skin as you visualize it, now Touch the tops the of hairs of your skin, as lightly as you would to feel only the drum skin's peak vibrations.

Where it is easiest for you to touch skin with hair on it, first wash and dry your hands and that skin. Move your hand and fingers lightly across the tops of those hairs. Concentrate on touching only the tops of those hairs, not the skin below. Practice moving back and forth, and in circles, touching lightly and gliding smoothly and slowly. Along with the drum visualization, this should give you a good physical sense of how lightly to touch.

Could you feel the tickle and perhaps the coolness?

If one hand has a difficult time touching only the hairs and not the skin below, try using the other hand, as it may have a lighter touch. If the hairs are too short to avoid touching the skin below, that's okay. Attempting to touch only the hairs in that difficult case is still a great practice for learning how to touch very lightly.

Let's move to the next step. Lightly touch the top surface of the skin across the back of your hand and forearm. Lightly glide your hand and fingertips across the tip-top surface of the skin. Practice the slow back and forth, circles and swirl techniques with your palm and fingertips along your skin or clothing, until you can create the tickling sensation and possible coolness. You may feel the tickle radiate to your spine, or whole body.

Give the skin a break every once in a while, for a few minutes. Once you can create the tickle, try to sustain it for a few moments, the session is finished. The neurons from that area of your skin have learned enough from this CBi Touch lesson. The tickle may spread through your whole body, too, and linger for a few moments.

During the next session, practice adding a slight amount of pressure. Rather than only feeling the tickle that spreads out across the skin, your skin may also notice contact points where the fingers touch the skin, just barely registering enough for localized feeling.

You may also try holding the touching hand as still as possible, while it lightly touches the skin. We cannot hold the hand absolutely still, no matter how hard we try, due to the heartbeat, plus hands do not hold themselves perfectly still while suspended. The slight motion of a suspended hand is enough for a Touch Master to apply the Touch effectively.

Hopefully, those descriptions provide an idea of how lightly to touch the skin or clothing for this intrinsic Touch technique to work at the novice level.

Once you can feel the tickle and chill, congratulations! You have learned the basic CB Intrinsic Touch technique. Be prudent. Use this wisely; only with pain that no longer serves a purpose. We will cover that point many more times, throughout the entire book, since it is critically important for safety.

Application to Painful Areas

After a student sitting before me has successfully applied the Touch very slowly and lightly, I ask him for permission to apply the Touch to the area(s) that currently hurts.

Applying the Touch over clothing works well if the clothing is not too billowy. It needs to have some contact with the student's skin to convey the vibrations of the Touch through the material to the skin. Contact, not more pressure, is all that is required. Applying the Touch over jeans or a business shirt doesn't present much of a problem. Close-knit shirtsleeves would be better than billowy shirtsleeves.

I apply the CB Intrinsic Touch slowly and very lightly to a broad area that includes and surrounds the pain (either on the hair, skin or indirectly to the clothing or shoe, depending on the location of pain). I tell my student that his or her job is to relax, and to let me know as soon as the pain has either stopped or is reduced significantly. His telling me is the only way I can know when to stop applying the Touch. Once the pain stops, applying the Touch should stop for that session.

We are training the neurons to respond to the Touch by stopping pain. Since applying the Touch for too long can cause the neurons to fatigue, I apply the CBi Touch only until the pain has significantly reduced or stopped. The Touch feels so good, it's hard to stop, but to be effective, try to avoid stimulating the neurons too much.

If a student can easily touch their painful area, on perhaps an arm, knee or hip, I will first demonstrate how to apply the Touch over his clothing, and before the pain disappears, let him try out his new skills on his own. Students are surprised at how quickly they find success.

For novice students applying the Touch for the first time, success for stopping pain usually takes a few minutes. For a practiced student, it may take only one minute or just a few seconds. When someone applies the Touch for another, success can take a bit longer.

When I apply the Touch to an area that a student cannot reach, perhaps to the middle of the back, after about 15 minutes I remind him that his job is to remain relaxed and to tell me when the pain stops.

My adult students often laugh, saying that the pain stopped a while ago. I ask why they didn't tell me sooner, and they'll say it's because the Touch feels so good, they don't want me to stop! It is a pleasant feeling, but we need to train the neurons to stop pain quickly, rather than confusing them (if that's possible) by emphasizing the pleasant feeling, instead of stopping once the pain has reduced or stopped - the desired outcome.

Fifteen to eighteen minutes should be the maximum limit for attempting to have a successful session. Let the skin reset for several minutes before trying again. Stop as soon as the Touch successfully controls the pain. Success is a personal judgment call. Everyone is different and each will learn their own ranges, limits (from reduction to stopping it), and preferences.

If my student says the pain is not stopping, it could mean the skin has fatigued or that the skin is not clean. We will take a break for several minutes while he washes and dries the underlying skin to make sure it didn't have interfering salt residue or perspiration causing drag. We try again a little later.

Also, we apply the Touch to more than just the 'spot' that hurts. Lightly touch the surface area where it hurts, plus at least another five-inch radius surrounding the hurt. Let's say there is a painful muscle near the elbow. Apply the Touch all around the forearm, elbow area and up toward the shoulder. If shoulder pain is stubborn, try applying the Touch to the skin or shirt, from the shoulder, all the way to the spine, rising up the neck and down the to include about one third of the spine, across and below the shoulder blades, back up to the shoulders and out the arms toward the elbows. You are activating all the light touch neurons you can to overcome the pain signals at the spinal cord. It's okay to overwhelm the pain neurons.

My reasoning for this is there are more pain neurons in the skin per square inch than there are light touch neurons. By touching a broader area surrounding the active pain neurons, our intention is to recruit as many painkilling light touch neurons as possible to sufficiently outnumber and overwhelm the pain-creating neurons.

After I spend a few moments showing a student how to apply the Touch to their actively painful area, occasionally their pain stops immediately and abruptly. We wait for a while to see if that pain will return, so the student can practice. If the pain doesn't return, the session is over. Sometimes he may have a different area that suddenly becomes painful. He can use that area for practicing the Touch, along with my guidance.

Pain can travel. Perhaps the pain was in the shoulder and nowhere else for days. However, when the Touch stops the shoulder pain, the arm may begin to hurt. Students then apply the Touch to the arm to make that new pain stop. Sometimes, then their wrist will hurt. That is normal. Simply follow or 'chase' the pain as it travels, applying the Touch wherever it is needed next.

We have found that, just as it works for me to control chronic pain for a student while I instruct him, this is also effective for caregivers or practitioners wanting to help their patients.

The caregiver first becomes one of my students, or reads this book, to correctly learn the skills. Then they apply the Touch for their patients, possibly also training the patients to apply the Touch for themselves. Or for a loved one who is unable to apply the Touch, a family member may learn how to apply the Touch for him. These skills become an act of love.

For the reader, once you are able to apply the CBi Touch to the tops of hairs, and then the skin on the back of your hand and forearm correctly, apply it to the areas that are hurting. Apply it slowly, gently, and lightly, avoiding weight or pressure. Apply it to the skin directly, or over clothing, bandages or an ice pack.

If you apply it over bandages or an ice pack, do not increase the pressure very much to compensate. The pain control neurons we stimulate respond to very light vibrations, and those vibrations can go through an ice pack. Your fingers do not need to touch the skin. This defies logic, but faint vibrations can do the trick.

To give a real-life example for how amazingly light the touch can be and still work, during my recovery from total knee replacement surgery, I applied the Touch lightly to the ice pack that was on top of my bandages. I did not press firmly to compensate for the thickness of the ice pack and bandages. I applied the Touch to the ice pack as if it were my skin (not hairs), with slight-pressure swirls. My knee could not 'feel' the Touch, while enough vibrations were transmitted all the way through the ice pack and bandages to stop pain during physical therapy. The correct touch neurons were activated, and they stopped the sensations of pain, so I could power through therapy. It's difficult to imagine the Touch working any more lightly than that.

What do I mean by light or faint vibrations? Visualize this by thinking of the tiny ridges on our fingertips (which create our fingerprints) as being microscopic wash boards. Dragging a stick rapidly across a real wash board will cause banging and vibrations. Stroking skin or clothing lightly with our fingertips causes very light, minuscule washboard vibrations.

When we talk about structures as tiny as nerve endings within the skin, think at the microscopic level to better understand their microscopic world. The neurons that we want to stimulate for mimicking imminent danger respond to super light vibrations.

As soon as weight is applied, they stop responding because, quite literally, weight does not activate them. Weight activates other touch neurons that let us know something with weight is touching us. That makes sense. Something with normal weight does not usually set off imminent danger alarms, at least not as much as a spider will. Rubbing a stubbed toe applies weight and that works for a stubbed toe, but it cannot work for chronic pain. Neurons responding to higher pressure are the wrong neurons for stopping chronic pain.

Sometimes the CBi Touch stops a novice's pain with our very first try, the very first pass or stroke. At other times, novices only reduce, rather than stop their pain with our first efforts over several minutes. They have significant reduction in painful sensations, yet they seem to be disappointed. Practice improves that.

This initial, limited success may be because the neurons in the skin are just waking up to their new role. With practice, full success is reached. Sharp pain tends to stop completely. The deep, dull pains tend to be stubborn. Even though it may take intermittent practice for 3 days, chronic (or acute) deep, dull pains will stop. Be patient and persistent. Practice the CBi Touch for a few minutes, perhaps three times a day for stubborn, deep pain. Success depends entirely on the individual's skill, the condition, their specific nervous system, and possible complications from medications.

Chronic pain may remain silent for several days following successful application of the Touch; perhaps even a week. By the time a student can make his pain remain silent for one week, the next time he applies the Touch, the pain may remain silent for several weeks to months.

I have mastered these techniques, so now normal acute pain, followed by no pain as tissues heal has replaced my chronic pain. I only need to deal with new injuries or conditions as they arise. Then, my pains remain silent for days, weeks, and months to years, depending on the individual causes for the pain. And they no longer become chronic. The same will hopefully be true for practiced students as they master these skills.

If an itch comes back after scratching it, without becoming frustrated, angry, analyzing it, or even thinking about it, we scratch it again. If chronic pain comes back, Touching can work in the same way.

Whenever chronic pain unfortunately comes back, or when persistent acute pain that is being controlled returns, merely CBi Touch it again. It's no big deal. It will take less time to successfully control the pain each time it comes back. Skills will progress from taking minutes to taking only moments for success. It will progress from needing circles and swirls to needing only one very light pass or brush across the skin (or clothing or shoe). Eventually, merely resting the hand lightly across that area will be sufficient.

Remember, these skills are only intended for chronic pain or diagnosed acute pain with a doctor's permission. Allow and endure acute pain until a doctor has made the diagnosis and s/he says that it is okay to practice CBi pain control techniques for this particular condition.

The Touch does not work for sudden or recurring spikes of acute pain, like when a nurse pulls out incision staples. It works best on pain that 'lingers' around long enough for the Touch to be applied and take effect.

Also, the various types of neurons that are involved in the pain control process must be healthy enough to fully participate in order for the Touch to work.

Resting my hand lightly across my toes on my shoe was what I caught myself doing when I first discovered the Touch. It did not need swirls or a brush because I had been doing the Touch for some months, long before I first caught myself doing it. I only used my relatively still hand. That faint, vibrational Touch stopped my foot's pain, and that was how I could walk in regular shoes without feeling pain for hours. Neuroplasticity healed my chronic pain because my neurons learned normal signaling patterns again. That allowed me to walk in flat shoes, and even barefooted, as much as I wanted.

These extraordinary skills became my new ordinary.

Effective Pressures

Thinking back to our scenarios of situations that take priority over pain, we decided the easiest way to trick the brain is to mimic imminent danger feelings. Examples could be faint touches caused by a mosquito, spider, chipmunk fur, or a slithering snake barely touching the skin. The touch of a mosquito is obviously very different from that of a snake slithering against the skin, which gives us the pressure range for effectively imitating a brush with imminent danger.

First, be the *mosquito*. Apply essentially no pressure to hairs above the skin while moving your fingers in circles or stroking back and forth. Never feel the weight of your fingers on the skin. This lightest pressure should result in feelings of coolness and a tickle, without the skin registering the fingers touching it. To understand what I mean, stroke only the hairs on the head, arm, or leg, without touching the scalp or skin. You'll feel a tickling sensation, yet not be able to specifically tell where the touching is actually occurring. The tickle feels generalized, without a specific location.

Next, be the *spider*. Change from touching only the hairs to also barely touching the skin. There is no 'weight' from your fingers, and you feel the tickle and coolness. The skin can't quite discern that fingertips are touching it, and the location of contact still feels generalized and nonspecific. (This is the lightest touch to use with an ice pack and bandages.)

Apply slightly more pressure to mimic the *chipmunk*. The skin registers that the fingers are touching it, but the fingers are not feeling the details of the skin beneath them. It's difficult to describe in words. This does not create the coolness and tickle, but it still works well.

Next, imitate a slithering *snake* by applying a tad more pressure. The pressure is still faint enough that it does not qualify as 'weight'. Your fingers just barely register what the skin feels like underneath as they touch it. That is close to the slight pressure I was applying to my shoe, when I first became aware of the Touch, back in 2010. There is no tickle or coolness, but it is still a light, vibrational touch. (This is the most pressure applied to an ice pack.)

If you have been trying for a while, and the Touch hasn't worked yet, begin again by relearning the pressure range starting with a "very light" touch across the top of hairs and progress to the mid-range. If you are still not having success, instead of using fingers, try using this high-tech tool: a clean feather duster.

Using ostrich *feather plumes* is an effective way to perform the Touch, especially if they provide the best way to touch painful areas that your hands cannot reach (middle of the back). Remember, move slowly and lightly.

Use the fluffy tips of the feathers, not the sides or scratchy shafts or quills. The scratch that the shafts or quills create activates the wrong neurons in the skin. Neurons that respond to scratching will not control pain.

So that prickly shafts won't interfere with the gliding process of the Touch, I trim shafts back by about an inch, preserving the fluffiness of the plumes. Stroking the tips of the feather duster plumes lightly and slowly across the surface of clothing or the skin is surprisingly effective.

Some students sound concerned when they say they cannot feel the feathers touching them, especially over their clothing. I ask if they noticed a tickle or chill. They are surprised to realize that they did. The tickle is all that matters. If you can't feel the feathers touching, look closely to see that they are touching; you might need to use a mirror to see it on your back. If you would prefer to feel the feathers, press a bit more firmly, but feeling the tickle is primary. It's an art worth perfecting.

That helps us understand the full range of pressures to apply during a glide, swirl, brush, or stroke in order to create the right vibrations for the CBi Touch to work (mosquito to spider to chipmunk to slithering snake).

CBi Touch Pressure Range Summary

1) *The Mosquito* – freshly washed and dried hand(s) gliding across the tops of hairs, like a mosquito, creating tickles and perhaps a cool sensation.

2) *The Spider* – add a tad more pressure, so the hand only slightly touches the skin, like a spider, with tickles and a chill.

3) *The Chipmunk* – add a bit more pressure so the coolness and tickles aren't there, but the touch is still weightless. The fingers register that they are touching the skin, but they aren't 'trying to feel' the skin. The skin registers that it is being touch, as if fur has lightly touched it, but the exact location of the touch and what is touching it is not discernible or clear.

4) *The Snake* – add a bit more pressure so the fingers can feel the skin, but just barely. It's barely enough to dampen the sound of a drum. The skin knows where it is being touched, as it might notice the scaly, slimy glide of a snake. Move slowly, softly.

5) *Feather Plumes* – use a feather duster for pains that are difficult to reach (trim prickly shafts back by about an inch). Notice the tickle or an eerie feeling. This is a great substitute for 'heavy' hands and a great tool for chronic pain control in general.

6) Applying actual pressure or weight to sooth, feel, rub, or caress the skin is out of range, because those kinds of touch do not activate the right neurons for chronic pain control.

Practice It to Perfect It

Rather than planning to practice the Touch when it is more convenient, practice it the moment chronic pain returns, just as you would scratch an itch. By practicing the Touch consistently, the nervous system will learn this is the desired response. It will eventually reduce chronic pain on its own, without coaxing. New pains will arise, but these neurons can be trained to identify and stop new chronic pain often before or seconds after you first notice pain. The need to apply the Touch will occur less and less often for that particular area. By applying the CBi Touch, the nervous system is actually 'unlearning' chronic pain. It is relearning how to be normal.

If you are not able to reach the painful area, even with a feather duster, ask for help from a significant other, friend or caregiver. Success with the Touch applied by others takes longer at first because your nervous system processes their touch differently. It might take one minute for you to control pain for yourself, while for a caregiver, it may take 10 -15 minutes at first to achieve the same result. Your skin should learn to recognize the other person's touch with continued practice, allowing the skills to improve and take effect sooner. Everyone is different. Give it time, maintain hope, and practice whenever the pain returns.

One of my chronic pain control students had diabetic neuropathy pain in her feet. Her significant other applied the Touch to one foot for 15 minutes during their first attempt before that foot's pain would stop. They used her other foot as a control by not applying the Touch to it. Her first foot remained pain-free for five hours, while pain from her control foot continued non-stop.

As with my diabetic student and her significant other, when I teach a student, it can take me 10 minutes or more for significant results, and I have practiced this for a long time. If the person helping you is new to this, they need time to learn how, and your clean skin must adjust to their touch. If it takes them 15 minutes, that is fine. That time interval should shorten with practice. If the skin fatigues, take a break, and try again a little later.

Pain serves a vital purpose. Seek help whenever its warranted. Endure new acute pain until a diagnosis is complete. Only stop pain that no longer serves a purpose.

Lack of pain, due to controlling it, does not mean something is cured or healed, or that there is no longer a need for concern. If pain has been silenced, it can't alert us any longer, so we must watch for other indications that an injury or condition is worsening, and then act responsibly. Our vigilance takes the place of pain. Do not let the lack of pain fool you. We do not want to inadvertently become our own cause for more harm.

Based on what is happening at an injury site with silenced pain, I remember to take the place of the 'missing' pain by being observant, checking for signs of worsening conditions, becoming alarmed despite not feeling pain, and quickly taking appropriate action. Remember to routinely follow up on your condition, with X-rays, etc., as you would if it were still painful.

Specific Touch Applications
(Use only against pains that no longer serve a purpose.)

Abdominal Pain ~

Wash and dry to remove salty perspiration residues for enhancing the tickles, if necessary. Apply the mosquito or spider pressure range, slowly swirling, using the fingers of both hands, on bare skin, covering the entire abdomen or tummy. The technique is correctly applied if chills and intense tickles are felt. (See Internal Organ Pain, p. 82.)

Fingernail or Toenail Removal ~

Apply the mosquito pressure range to the full length of the toe or finger, starting on the foot or hand, while being careful to not touch the open wound. If there is a bandage, apply the Touch slowly and lightly over the bandage, too. It works best to stroke in one direction, from the foot or hand, toward and past the toe or finger.

Foot Pain ~

To a clean, dry foot with clean, dry hands, double swirling in the mosquito or spider range is best, covering the entire foot, ankle, and calf. Applying the Touch with a feather duster works very well, especially when the foot is hard to reach.

For long-term chronic pain of the foot, eventually the chipmunk range or lightly resting the hand on the skin or shoe may work, as the nervous system adapts to its new role for pain control. In my case, my chronic pain eventually stopped (practicing from 2010-2014).

Furry Pet's Pain ~

For your pet's arthritic pain, and other chronic pain issues, training with the Touch can work wonders to control their pain, without the fog from pain medicine.

Begin his/her training using the mosquito or mouse to see if your pet tolerates the tickling. My cat couldn't at first. He would hiss and threaten me when we began trying the Touch for his arthritic back and joints. I persisted, ignoring his threats, until finally he got it.

I knew the Touch worked on him immediately because his limping would stop and not return for hours. Eventually the pain was gone for weeks to months, as his nervous system learned to respond to the Touch.

After many weeks of training, he stopped resisting my help. He realized he needed to endure the tickle to get his pain to stop. It became very matter-of-fact for him. He needed to be standing, and not in my lap.

He used to grimace while he allowed me to apply the Touch. He would remain still, taking a step or two to see if the pain had stopped. He'd stay if he needed more strokes of the Touch, and would move on once his pain had stopped. He wouldn't be limping and was visibly happy once the pain stopped each time.

After about two years of using the Touch, he became a Touch Master. He would park himself in front of me, facing forward. It would finally dawn on me that he was asking for the Touch. I would position my thumbs above his neck, near his shoulders, and position my fingers so they lightly cover his shoulders and throat. He'd walk slowly forward until my hands met his tail and pause.

80

If he needed more strokes for the pain to stop, he waited for me to step forward, reposition my hands near his neck and shoulders, and then he would again walk slowly forward again, in effect performing the Touch himself, knowing my hands would remain in position, touching lightly enough to apply it in the mosquito - mouse range, repeating this process until his pain stopped. Once the pain had stopped, he'd move on to the next thing he needed to get done for the day, like take a nap. He relied on and used the Touch for years.

Touch the top of your animal's fur or hair, stroking with the grain, so to speak, using mosquito - mouse range, continuing until the pet lets you know the pain has stopped. It could take 3 - 8 strokes. My cat and I hope this will help your pets, too.

Hip Pain ~

For severe, intractable hip pain that does not seem to respond to the Touch, modifications in the timing for applying the Touch can work wonders. Apply the Touch at night, immediately before going to bed. Apply it slowly and lightly, covering as much skin as possible from the waistline to the ankle, surrounding the entire leg. A feather duster may make it easier to reach areas that are difficult to Touch otherwise.

Then sleep for several hours before getting up, giving the hip tissues and the nervous system the extra time needed to execute control over extreme pain conditions. Pain control can remain in effect until late in the afternoon the following day. Severe hip injury is so hard.

Touch techniques do not address the extreme emotional depression that may accompany an extremely injured or eroded hip. Use MBPC (Part III) to help your psyche maintain distance from negative emotions. It's easy to get pulled down from the depression injured hips can induce. Dismiss the mind's attempts to make you believe it's all over. That's just mind stuff. Reject it and breathe in life. Do not fear hip repair - save your life.

Internal Organ Pain ~

As with painful bones, connective tissues and muscles, organ pain is addressed by applying the Touch to the surrounding skin above the painful organ. Touch a broad area surrounding the pain lightly. It may be necessary to include touching along the spine, above and below the organ. Using a feather duster may help.

For organs in the front lower abdominal area, include Touching one or both thighs, extending the Touch up to the waistline. For organs in the upper abdominal area, include one or both shoulders and neck. Include the back, directly behind the organ, from that side to spine.

Applying the Touch to 'more than enough' skin is best until you discover the specific areas that are essential to Touch for your specific condition. The goal is to recruit more than enough light touch neurons to block all of the organ's pain signals when the neurons compete at the spinal cord.

Use the mosquito through spider pressure range on clean, bare skin or over clothing. Touching the skin directly is best for organs, depending on skill level, etc.

Knee Pain ~

The general rule applies to knees - apply the mosquito to chipmunk range, using double swirls with the fingers of both hands, on either the skin, jeans, bandages, covering an area all the way around the knee, including the area 5 or 6 inches above and below. Eventually resting the hand lightly or a single swipe at chipmunk pressure will be enough to stop the pain.

Low Back Pain ~

With clothing on or clean, bare skin, using either the back of the hands, or fingers, whatever is comfortable/possible, at spider or chipmunk pressures, swirl an area that includes the painful area, plus a 5- or 6-inch radius, 12-inch diameter. If pain radiates down to the hip or leg, include those areas, too, including the expanded radius, as needed for those areas. Touching more than enough skin is more effective than not Touching enough.

Middle Back Pain ~

A clean feather duster works best for the middle to upper back. Try to use only the fluffy ends of ostrich feathers on clean bare skin, or over clothing that is not too billowy. Use a mirror if possible, to make sure the feathers are touching the shirt or skin. Notice the traveling tickle to gauge success. It is not necessary to 'feel' the stroking of the feathers themselves - concentrate mostly on feeling a faint, radiating tickle and chill.

Migraine Headaches ~

Migraine pain is often the easiest to stop. If the migraine involves the face and head, apply the Touch to both areas. This should resolve the migraine very quickly, again and again, whenever necessary. If the migraine comes back, apply these technique again.

For migraines that involve the scalp, use the mosquito to spider range and Touch only the tops of hairs. Rarely go down into the hair. Prioritize grazing the top, trying to make it feel as if an insect is walking across your hair.

For migraines that include the forehead, eyes, or cheekbones, use the spider pressure range, touching the skin only with the fingertips and use swirls. Move slowly and ever so lightly. Include touching the hairs.

The Touch does not alleviate nausea, a sudden drop in energy level, or light sensitivity. It may still be necessary to lie flat and take the day off. The Touch does not affect the aura, nor temporary blindness. The upside is, since the pain is gone, auras are more fun to watch. Do not drive while experiencing an aura. Pull off to the side of the road.

Neck Pain ~

Apply the Touch in the mosquito to chipmunk range. Include the entire neck, lower portion of the head and face. Continue the Touch down the neck toward the middle back, out to the edge of the shoulders, and/or to the upper chest. If only one side of the neck hurts, it may work well to address only that one side, but test continuing out to the other side, at least a little bit.

Using a feather duster works great for the neck. It may make reaching the back of the neck, between the shoulder blades and out to the backs of the shoulders much easier. A caregiver might help by applying the Touch with hands or feather duster on clean, bare skin or on top of a shirt.

Nose Surgery Pain ~

The Touch is very effective with nose surgery recovery pain. Touch very lightly over the bandages, lightly and slowly across the eyelids, down the cheeks, across the lips and chin. Brush lightly and slowly across the forehead. It may surprise you how painless the recovery can be, using the Touch. Unfortunately, the Touch will not help with nausea. Anti-nausea pills are a great help.

Shoulder Pain ~

Apply the Touch for shoulder pain using the mosquito to spider range. Using a feather duster will be a tremendous help. Touch all around the shoulder, across the back of the neck, up to the scalp, down the spine about 1/2 way, down the chest, out about 5 inches on each side, down and all around the arm, even past the elbow. Less area may be needed the next time.

Spinal Nerve Pain ~

Sparking pins and needles pain, or shooting, burning pain that has no visible source, yet seems to be in very specific, discrete locations, and rarely changes its tune, may point to a pinched spinal nerve condition.

For example, if the pain hurts in a very specific spot under the scapula, or in a muscle near the elbow, but nothing has happened to the elbow or scapula, plus the skin is not red or swollen, and there are no signs of injury, presume there is a pinched spinal nerve for intrinsic pain control purposes. Get a valid diagnosis.

Only after a proper diagnosis, apply the Touch using the mosquito to spider range, on clothing or clean, bare skin. Use swirls with the fingers or the fluffs of a feather duster. Apply the Touch to the places that hurt and expand that area to include a 5- to 6-inch-wide path all the way back to and surrounding the spine.

Deep, strong, and powerful spinal nerve or spinal cord pain can be very stubborn. Use the Touch perhaps 3 or 4 times a day, even if the pain does not lessen. It takes stubborn nerve or cord pain time to surrender to the Touch. Also apply any of the ten MBPC techniques that work with your situation. The Touch might work the first day or it might take three days, but it will work, unless the erosion or spinal compression is so great that the pain is warning of severe damage. The doctor may suggest surgery.

Along with spinal nerve or cord involvement comes the risk for long-term loss-of-function, and even permanent muscle weakness or paralysis. Do not risk incontinence. Do not mess around. Act quickly.

Surgery Recovery Pain ~
Underneath the ice pack and bandages that have not yet been removed, lies the skin surrounding the incision. To make the incision, and while performing the surgery,

some of the nerves were unavoidably cut. Consequently, some of the skin may now feel numb. That is normal following surgery, and it is okay. Over time, some of the sensation will return, but for now, the skin may be completely numb in large or small areas.

Therefore, a few of the neurons we use for the Touch may not be able to respond because they have been disconnected, so to speak. So, the Touch may need to be applied to a much wider area for enough light touch neurons to be activated. And, just because an area is numb, we can't be sure if the light touch neurons are equally numb. It's a matter of trial and error because every patch of skin has a different story.

Once the bandages are removed and you can touch the skin directly for the first time, the outline of numbness will become more obvious.

Apply the Touch to the skin close to the incision (which may be numb) and to the surrounding areas that are numb, attempting to feel the tickle and chill to see if any light touch neurons are 'awake'. Make note of where the touch neurons respond and continue to include those areas when you apply the Touch.

Also apply the Touch to the surrounding areas that are not numb. Remember to include the 5-inch minimum radius surrounding the painful area when you apply the Touch. The WDRs at the spinal cord will hopefully receive enough stimulation from light touch neurons to counter the pain. Application of the Touch tends to work out just fine fairly soon following surgery.

Trigeminal Nerve Pain ~

Even though the Trigeminal Nerve is the most painful cranial nerve, it is surprisingly easy to tame. The trigeminal can be as fierce as a great lion or tiger, but it tames as easily as a kitten.

Just because the pain is excruciating does not mean it will take a long time for the Touch to work. The pain can stop in a moment or seconds. If it takes longer, no big deal; it will take less time with more practice.

Mosquito through spider pressure range. Clean, dry hands and skin. Use faint fingertip swirls or lightly brushing in one direction. A single, spider-light swipe might be enough. Follow the same 5- to 6-inch radius rule to be included in the Touch area.

For screaming, painful eyes - touch as lightly as a mosquito to slowly brush and swirl the eyelids and surrounding skin with the fingertips.

For painful jaw, nose, parotid glands - mosquito-light, slow brush and swirls where it hurts and the surrounding skin.

For dental, adenoidectomy, tonsillectomy, uvulectomy, surgery recoveries - mosquito-light, slow strokes with fingertips straight down the cheeks, jaw line, under the chin and down the neck. Notice how each acute pain spike from swallowing will end surprisingly quickly, too. Breathing will not cause as much pain, if any.

Successes with CB Intrinsic Touch

Pins and needles, sharp, burning
Torn ligament, tendon, cartilage
Interstitial cystitis pain relief
Deviated septum sinus pain
Diabetic neuropathic pain
Trigeminal neuralgia pain
Any Surgery recovery
Migraine headaches
Deep, grinding pain
Cystic fibrosis pain
Sciatic nerve pain
Muscle cramping
Neurogenic pain
Abdominal pain
Meniscus pain
Deep bruising
Flu shot ache
Fibromyalgia
Broken bone
Spinal nerve
Lower back
Headaches
Mild burns
Old injury
Arthritis
Sprains
Strains
Aches

Part III

CB INTRINSIC MINDFULNESS-BASED PAIN CONTROL

Matter Over Mind

How we use the mind matters.

Adults can control chronic pain for hours, days, or weeks at a time following the application of the CB Intrinsic Touch. Combining CBi Touch with Mindfulness-based Pain Control (MBPC) techniques can result in long-term, and sometimes automatic control over or recovery from chronic pain. MBPC amplifies and expands the power of the Touch.

Relying on MBPC techniques has become second nature for my mind. They lessen lingering pain as it occurs. MBPC continues to run silently in the background, without my having to think about it.

Since 2014, I have not suffered chronic pain from my permanently injured foot, nor have I needed to protect it at night from the weight of bed sheets or covers. I can walk barefooted, in slippers or use flat street shoes. I can even comfortably wear hiking boots. I give full credit to applying the CBi Touch initially, followed by MBPC, which runs continuously, effortlessly.

Over the past few years, my nervous system learned to be proactive against initiating chronic pain, apparently ever again. Acute pain works normally in my foot now, as it did before my injury. It sometimes gets re-injured, hurts, and heals while its new acute pain stops very quickly, due to MBPC. The foot's ligaments are still damaged, but its pain processes have normalized.

You may find that some situations need a jump start with the Touch, while others respond just fine with mental MBPC techniques administered alone. They usually work phenomenally well when applied together.

The bottom line is practicing MBPC with the CBi Touch teaches the mind to ignore specific chronic pain signals. "If you don't use them, you will lose them" applies. Chronic pain is good to lose.

Other chronic pain issues have occurred for me since 2010. The Touch and MBPC have taken care of all of them. As described earlier, regaining muscle function for my muscles, which had been weakened by bulging discs and pinched spinal nerves in my back, occurred only days following application of the Touch, along with MBPC constantly running in the background.

I study current research articles that help me understand how these techniques work. I earned my master's degree (Anatomy/Biomedical Science, 2001) studying neurobiology at Colorado State University, so I understand the research findings. To understand how the MBPC techniques work so effectively, I reviewed current cognitive neuroscience research. I am able to apply the current pain related research findings to virtually all of the CBi techniques in support of their effectiveness. I won't delve too deeply into pain science with this book. But including some pain science is helpful because with the knowledge and understanding that I share with you comes Power. Controlling pain requires empowerment.

Knowledge and understanding help us feel more comfortable about new ideas, which helps enable us to reach the state of mind necessary for profound, long-term, automatic control of chronic pain.

Because the nervous system amplifies and sustains pain, the instinctive mind may presume it knows better than what it reads in this book. It may stubbornly try to undermine change and thwart any chance for success at controlling pain. Some understanding of the pain process at the cellular level provides the strength we need to counter the instinctive mind's objections in order to improve our chances for gaining control over pain. We are not 'blocking' pain. We are controlling it.

Also, we must delve into pain science a little bit so I can communicate and describe MBPC techniques more effectively. Knowing more about the science will increase the reader's understanding about how the nervous system creates and stops pain. The science helps us understand how to influence the mind's priorities, emotions, behaviors, and thoughts in order to gain control over chronic pain.

To control chronic pain for the long-term, along with the potential to achieve some degree of return of function for muscles or glands, stepping beyond the ordinary is required.

As mentioned in the Preface, our choices are between following ordinary beliefs or taking a chance on the truly extraordinary to break down barriers and make real progress. It is nice to know that science backs up these extraordinary techniques for chronic pain control.

Emergent Properties

Without going too deeply into neurobiology, we benefit from knowing something about the nervous system. Neurons are the main types of cells that make the nervous system work. They are in the nerves that span the distance from the fingertips or toes, all the way to the spinal cord. Neurons are also in the spinal cord and the brain. There are about as many neurons in the gut as there are in the spinal cord. Some neurons in the brain are so tiny, an estimated 30,000 brain neurons would fit inside the head of a straight pin. It is difficult to imagine how small those neurons are.

When we look inside neurons at the nanometer level, $1x10^{-9}$ meter, we realize they are made of ions, atoms, and molecules, which interact with each other according to the laws of physics. Their interactions are dynamic, predictable, and are understood exquisitely well. Their complexities are incredible at the individual level, and colossally incredible when we consider what they can do collectively, as a system.

At the micro level, neurons are arranged to communicate with each other within specific groupings or pathways. Neuronal pathways determine which predictable thoughts, emotions, feelings and behaviors are expressed by an individual. Within a pathway, neurons interact or communicate with each other, from one neuron to the next and the next. Each neuron may communicate with thousands of neurons at a time.

Through the default factory settings of the brain, it takes only microseconds for neural pathways at the micro level to create perceptions, thoughts, emotions, and behaviors at the macro level. This is the function of the brain, which results in an amazing emergent property – the mind. The mind is very mysterious.

There is truly nothing solid about the mind; we cannot touch the mind, as we can touch an arm or a leg. And the brain-created mind, with its perceptions, thoughts, and emotions, becomes who we think we are.

No one yet understands how consciousness or the mind arises out of the ions, atoms, and molecules, or from the neurons and other cells of the brain. Even though we understand the physics behind how the molecules of cells interact, along with the energies involved in order for them to function, and we understand the mechanics of the chemistry that creates the biology, we still cannot account for how the mysterious synergies occurring between all the components, along with the energies of the brain, result in their emergent properties - thoughts, consciousness, and the mind. It is a grand example of synergy at work; the total effect from the parts working together is significantly greater than the sum of each part's contribution alone. Consciousness and the mind hold exquisite mysteries and forever offer new frontiers.

Aside from not knowing how consciousness or even thoughts arise, the mind is fairly predictable. We can work with what is understood so far. We know the mind can learn and change. Controlling our perspectives can change default settings for thoughts and behaviors, which then alter the pathways in the brain; neuroplasticity. Neuroplasticity restructures the brain and transforms the mind. Neuroplasticity leads to altering our subjective reality, the reality our mind creates for us, which we each experience as our individual, unique world. An interesting fact is, pain is just as real as no pain, and neither one is 'solid'. The fact that pain is part of the mind means we are fortunately able to reconstruct our mind's reality about pain, too.

When new habits become second nature, we have altered neuronal pathways at the cellular level within the brain. Due to continued practice over time, the new pathways became the preferred settings of the brain, and a new version of the mind exists.

Think about how practicing the piano over time has the potential to transform someone from one who could not play the piano into a person with the mind of a concert pianist. For our purposes, this is how practicing mindfulness changes the structure of the brain, which changes how we experience life at the deepest levels. It changes us from someone under the control of chronic pain into a master who controls chronic pain, and possibly restores normal pain processing.

When we change how we choose to think, we can indirectly change which neurons communicate with each other. With continued practice, we can change neuronal preferences, and create new pathways (novice pianist to concert pianist). If we transform from being reactive to being responsive toward pain, we can cause new preferences or pathways to form, which then create new comfort zones over time. In that way, we get entirely new results. The potential for this type of changeability or the neuroplasticity within the nervous system is what makes long-term control of chronic pain possible.

The brain is capable of incredible change, but as to being successful, we must have intention. Intention implies we are committed to practicing change on purpose. Otherwise, the brain will continue to repeat the same old stuff, and chronic pain will continue because, at the basic level, brains do not like to change.

With practice, the more we use intentionally preferred thought patterns, the stronger those new preferences become. It's stubborn, but the brain will comply.

For advantageous change, we apply the axiom "the more you use it, the stronger it gets." For the old pathways and thoughts that we want to use less often, we apply the axiom "if you don't use it, you'll lose it."

As with many things about the mind, we can apply these concepts to the perceptions of pain. What is the opposite of chronic pain? The opposite is less or no chronic pain, with the potential to reset normal patterns.

Brain response times are faster for repetitious thoughts and reactions, just as water reacting to gravity flows more freely down a steeper hill. Water will follow the same path. The ruts get deeper, making those ruts more preferred. Neurons also prefer using the same old pathways, the paths of least resistance.

It takes energy to make water follow a different path. Likewise, it takes energy or work to encourage neurons to leave their old rut to form their new comfort zone.

Through mindfulness and intention, by watching our mind and taking the time to choose a response, rather than simply reacting again and again, we supply the energy and necessary conditions for nurturing the formation of new neural pathways. That is how we produce new comfort zones for the brain, and its mind. That is how we alter our reality to experience pain differently. We just need to know which new responses to substitute the for old reactions, and how to apply those responses correctly, efficiently, and effectively.

While developing new pathways, response times will be slow at first. With practice, once the new pathways and comfort zones are fully established, response times become faster, potentially as fast as the reaction times of the old, reactive pathways.

Responsible and intentional changes in expressions of thoughts, emotions, and behaviors, plus changes in feelings (pain vs no pain via CBi Touch), together coax the brain into these new comfort zones. New preferences that feel better become second nature. Controlling chronic pain, rather than letting chronic pain be in control, becomes the new norm fairly quickly. Eventually, responding rather than reacting becomes second nature, and the old reactive, painful default, factory settings of the mind become the old paths traveled less often.

As with mind and thought, pain is not solid like an arm or a leg. Chronic pain is made of mind-stuff. If the mind learns how to stop using them, chronic pain pathways can truly be lost. If you don't use it, you lose it.

Pain Is Perception

The word 'pain' has different connotations. It can refer to negative emotional suffering due to some type of loss or to noxious physical suffering due to tissue damage, disease, pinched nerves, or any number of other physical and emotional conditions.

Noxious physical pain begins as simple on/off 'sensory information'. The information originates at the tissue level, perhaps due to a cut in the skin or injury to an organ. The information/signal travels inside sensory neurons within nerves to pass the information on to the pain pathways located in the spinal cord, which then pass their signals on to the brainstem pathways, and finally communication is made with neurons in specific areas of the brain responsible for pain perception. The information is modified at every step along the way.

Each set of neurons along the way modifies the very basic, binary on/off signals or sensory information coming to them from the injury site in precise and specific ways, eventually creating exquisitely precise, seemingly real perceptions of pain by the time all the information reaches to the cortex of the brain. By definition, physical pain hurts exactly like the injury or condition must seem to hurt.

Interpretation is the process of modification which adds very complex meaning to the initial, binary, on/off sensory signals. Interpretation specifies pain characteristics for intensity and type of pain, the emotional characteristics for how unpleasant or noxious the pain will feel, and details for the precise location of the injury. All characteristics for the pain are determined through the interpretation process.

Interpretation morphs into perception once the complete package of modified, interpreted information reaches various destination regions within the brain's cerebral cortex. Awareness of pain occurs simultaneously with perception, literally inside the cortex of the brain.

Perhaps the most important purpose and result of the interpretation process is to ensure the resulting pain perception makes pain seem objectively 'real', and that it unquestioningly exists at and originates from the injury site. Interpretation links the perception of pain so intimately with the injury that perception of pain and the real injury seem to be one.

Actually, the perception of pain occurs or exists only in specific regions of the cortex of the brain. The moment those regions give us pain perception is the same moment pain seems 'real', yet we are absolutely certain that the pain exists only at the injury site; wrong.

Pain perceptions emerge from, exist within, and are maintained and sustained only by the brain, as part of the mind, like thoughts. Tissues become injured somewhere in the body, but pain is resides within the brain. Pain is an emergent property of the brain and is experienced only by the mind. The mind's job is to convince us that pain exists at the injury site. The fact that pain seems 'solidly real' is instinctive and imperative for serving its purpose of ensuring our survival.

An injury site is objectively real in an empirically 'solid' way. A cut or burn can be seen, and its size can be measured. Pinched nerves can't be seen from the outside, but the condition can be verified, visualized, and measured empirically using MRI and X-ray. The brain associates physical pain with an objectively real injury site so seamlessly that we believe the two are one. Through its close association with the injury, pain disguises its truth under a façade of being as solid or as objectively real as the injury. Pain is not objectively real.

This is not someone's personal truth or belief. This is factual truth. This truth does not depend on where you were born, where you live, or what you believe. It does not depend on your culture or education. This is a solid, scientific fact: pain is not objectively real.

Not only do we instinctively equate pain with injury, we equate pain with harm. If you were to accidentally grab the hot handle of a frying pan with your bare hand, your hand would register the burn and instantly release the handle as you jump back.

Because the brain/mind equates the hurt of pain with harm, and the burning sensations continue in your hand, even though you successfully fled from the hot panhandle, your urge is to get the hurt off of your hand, or to flee from your hand, just as you fled from the hot handle. You may shake and flail the hand all around, trying to get away from its 'hurtful' pain, yet the perception of pain continues. You want to get away from the pain; you don't want it, you hate it. I exaggerated to make the point that we can't successfully flee from pain.

Pain can hurt a whole lot, yet except for the stress it causes, pain is not harming us, and it is not causing the tissue damage. That confuses the brain; the fact that I bring this point up may even be confusing.

We think the damage and its pain are one and the same, but pain is not causing further damage or injury. Pain is only initiated by whatever caused the injury. Pain is real within the brain, yet it is not creating more harm. Pain is not damaging the body. Pain is merely a perception of the mind. Pain is the mind's alarm system about the true damage, condition, or injury.

I do not like to use the phrase "it is all in your head" because of the negative connotations. I do not trivialize suffering. However, we need to analyze this because we need a paradigm shift. Pain is a real perception located in the head. Thoughts are real and they are in the head. A dream is real. Hunger is real. Joy is real. A lot of real and intangible things exist in the head, the brain, the mind.

Relying on our mind alone, no matter what else we do, except for utilizing research and education, we cannot perceive the true, objective reality that pain is the subjective, intangible end product of the nervous system's interpretation of pain signals, and that pain can only ever be in the brain. It is a powerful perception, yet still, only a figment of the mind.

We are tricked by the brain/mind for very good reasons. To be effective, pain and injury must seem to be solidly one. Getting help is the mind's primary objective and it uses a subjective trick to get what it needs. To overcome chronic pain, education helps us see its reality.

To control chronic pain completely and entirely, we must not only address it with the CBi Touch, from the bottom-up, but we must also address pain from within the brain and the mind, exactly where pain resides.

It takes education and knowledge to comprehend the truth about pain's intangible nature, plus mindfulness training for the tools and skills necessary to combat the instinctive pain settings of the mind. We can exert an amazing amount of power over pain, once we learn how to work with it directly, through the mind.

This is, perhaps, where some of the uncomfortable feelings accompanying the extraordinary come into play. Minds are powerful. We've heard that and realize at some level that we do not use our mind to its fullest potential. This is one of those instances. Controlling unnecessary or chronic pain by exercising more of the mind's hidden potential offers opportunities for expanding our mental capacity. Learning these skills is easily within our grasp.

Unlike learning to how to play the piano to become a concert pianist, learning how to utilize the mind's potential for controlling the pain it creates requires neither a natural gift nor a lot of time. Yet, exactly like becoming a concert pianist, it requires intention to provide the necessary energy, like moving water uphill, to get past the brain's objections to change, to work past our instinctive (erroneous) beliefs that pain is real and uncontrollable; it takes intention to release the subconscious attachments and protections we instinctively harbor for feeling and sustaining pain.

The paradigm shift is simple. We must allow facts to define the true substance and allow facts to describe the real matter that constitutes pain, in order for us to understand the true reality about pain. Then we prioritize that factual matter over the ordinary mind-stuff, over the instinctive beliefs that we harbor about pain, which the mind forces on us daily.

To better comprehend the matter, or the substance of pain, we need to learn more about what pain is, and more about the determining factors that contribute to how pain is created. With a deeper understanding, it becomes easier to recognize and overcome our instincts in order to control chronic pain by simply using the mind, literally, against its own mind-stuff.

The subjective nature of pain is the primary reason certain mindfulness techniques for controlling chronic pain are effective. There is usually more power within these techniques than within pain itself.

Welcome to the Extraordinary.

Subjective Reality

The fact that all pain is located within the brain, inside the head, is actually fortunate because that fact makes pain susceptible to the changing conditions of the mind. This makes pain fluid. This makes pain 'subjective'.

The Online dictionary at Dictionary.com lists its fourth and fifth definitions of subjectivity as "internal reality" and "relating to properties or specific conditions of the mind as distinguished from general or universal experience", respectively.

In support of this point about subjectivity, back when I was three or four years old, I was left alone to take showers by myself. Shampoo bottles were made of glass back then, and the tub was cast iron. To this day, I can clearly remember what happened. You can probably guess where I'm going with this.

The shampoo bottle sat at the far corner of the tub on a little ledge. As I picked up the bottle, it slipped through my wet, little hands and broke when it hit the hard surface of the tub. Glass and shampoo shattered and splattered in all directions at that end of the tub.

I stood there startled at first, and then my reaction became that of amazement. I noticed all the shiny glass pieces coated with creamy yellow shampoo lying on the floor of the tub. (Glass bottles were not tempered back then, so some of the broken pieces were very large and all were sharp.)

To an itty-bitty kid, the most attractive piece of glass was the biggest. It consisted of the circular bottom of the bottle along with a long vertical portion of its side. The vertical portion tapered to a point. It looked like a sparkly, glittery, glass knife with a bottle-bottom handle.

While leaning over to pick up that shiny piece of glass, red caught my eye. I noticed a wide-open gash in the inside calf of my right leg. I stared inside the gash, seeing the exposed muscle and the inside edges of the skin with a bumpy fat lining. I didn't feel pain from the wound until after I saw it, had a good, long look at it, and figured out what it was.

Then my screaming began. I was so scared. I wanted to get away, yet I remained frozen in place because I noticed all the glass pieces blocking any exit. I looked down and back to watch the blood mixing with the creamy yellow shampoo and shower water as they streamed together toward the drain. My father came to save me.

I was not concerned or in any pain until my mind realized there was an injury. That experience helps point out the fact that pain can be very subjective. Subjectivity depends on mental interpretations. Whether or not we actually perceive and feel pain depends on a lot of things.

The brain doesn't care if something is objectively or subjectively real. Our brain easily convinces us that when it says something is 'real', it is absolutely 'Real'. We tend to apply the same definition of 'real' to intangible, subjective, mind-stuff just as we apply 'real' to tangible objects or solid things, like tables or chairs.

For example, with chronic spinal nerve pain, the brain may tell us the 'injury' originates in an arm muscle, instead in the spine where the spinal nerve is being pinched. Pain tells us an injury is 'right there', highlighting a muscle that seems to be crying out in pain, and we believe that it is. We look and look at the 'injured muscle' site, but see absolutely no swelling, redness, or any other objective signs of injury on the skin. The mind pinpoints the pain so explicitly as being with the muscle, the physical injury MUST be there. The muscle has to be injured. When a doctor tells us it is not injured, that infuriates us. The disconnect lies with how the brain interprets pain signals and develops its perceptions of pain, which we choose to believe as solid, real evidence over whatever a doctor says is real.

The brain tricks us by disguising the *subjective* nature of pain as being objectively real, and by convincing us that pain is inseparably one with what must be an objective injury, even if the supposed injury is illusory.

In order to turn the tables and trick the brain, it is very important to realize pain truly and factually is a creation of, and it only ever exists within *the mind*. Finally realizing the facts helps us look more objectively at pain itself. To control it, we must address pain objectively. The mind can take advantage of its pain's fluid, subjective, mind-stuff nature. This is like pulling back the curtain to see the Wizard of Oz was only a man.

In a revolutionary way, we can control chronic pain because subjectivity depends on mental conditions. We can better take control of our mental conditions when we approach this with resolve and intention, which focus boundless energy on our intentional manipulation of the mind, and thus, more effectively control the subjective reality that the mind creates. Subjectivity allows us to, quite literally, use mental (mind) manipulation against the mind itself to eventually wipe many types of chronic pain right out of existence, as pain-related regions in the brain learn, or perhaps relearn, their role in pain control.

Pain is a real, yet subjective perception. Whether pain is acute or chronic, the brain links it to a location in the body and gives it the illusion of being one with the presumed tissues involved. Amazingly enough, the full experience of pain depends entirely on our current state of mind. For example, consider the two mental states, asleep versus awake, and how each handles pain differently. When we are awake, we feel pain. When we are asleep, we do not feel pain.

We are fortunate this is the case. Using different mental states provides us with loopholes to skirt around pain. Through greater understanding and intentional practice, we can combine the natural flexibility gained through subjectivity (which is very vulnerable to change), plus neuroplasticity (which helps neural pathways learn from and sustain this change) to alter whatever the mind decides is intangibly 'real'.

Since both types of feelings, pain and no pain, are conjured up by the mind, they are emergent properties of the mind. Feeling no pain is just as intangibly, subjectively 'real' as feeling pain. Through intelligent and intentional manipulations, we can change the mind's subjectively 'real' experience right now, from pain to no pain.

Is this 'mind over matter'? Not really. The opposite is true. It is more accurate to think of this as giving facts priority over mind-stuff, or 'matter over mind'.

Subjective pain is the 'mind', while the objective realities about pain constitute the 'matter'. Pain is created within certain regions of the brain where pain is intangible and subjective. The mind is the only thing that makes us 'think' pain is objective and real. It's not. Unlike mind over matter, using matter over mind works.

We do not need to spend any more time on futile attempts to force 'mind over matter' to work, or to believe 'mind over matter' should stop pain. That's the wrong perspective. The default setting of the mind does not care about whether or not its 'reality' is factually real. The mind believes it's right. But that is wrong. Facts matter more than mind-stuff.

Open your mind and loosen your attachments to believing whatever your mind tells you to believe. We can learn the facts about how the mind works. We can use the facts to figure out how to manipulate the mind to get it to fall in line with the matter (the facts), which actually matters the most. Given knowledge of the facts, the subjective and fluid nature of pain, and our ability to intelligently manipulate the mind, we have natural abilities for true, objective control over chronic pain.

Matter Triumphs Over Mind.

Neuroplasticity

The ability to create acute pain to accompany an injury is setup during the development of the nervous system in the womb. It is instinctive, normal, and beneficial. Acute pain creation is coupled with the nervous system's automatic pain 'control' pathways, which will end the creation of acute pain as tissues heal.

Unfortunately, some parts of the pain pathways are susceptible to abnormal change under certain conditions. When chronic pain results from abnormal changes within the nervous system, it happens after the full development of the pain pathways. Therefore, these new chronic pain pathways are not linked to an instinctive or automatic process to naturally end the pain. Sometimes, the ON switch is not correctly connected to an OFF switch anymore, hence pain becomes 'chronic'.

Or with other chronic pain conditions, the problem may be that acute pain returns too easily, over and over again, even after it has been stopped over and over again. The neurons that could end it may be injured or dormant. Pain pathways are complex, so scenarios are complex.

'Neuroplasticity' refers to the fact that certain types of neurons can alter their activity in response to these post-development changes in the neurons they communicate with. They can even reorganize their pathways. Changing activity levels and reorganizing pathways physically restructures the brain. These changes are physically measurable. They can alter mind-stuff. These changes can alter the reality of our mind-created world. We can intentionally direct this.

Perhaps addressing this from a different perspective would be helpful. When we consider the nervous system's pain pathways, it basically creates two normal pain states during development: the no-pain-state and the acute-pain-state. We are usually in the no-pain-state. In response to an injury or painful condition, the acute-pain-state is activated to feel pain now. Pain serves its vital purpose - alerting us to a new injury or condition, and pain helps us track the progress toward healing. The nervous system automatically returns to the no-pain-state as tissues heal, after acute pain's purpose has been served.

Due to abnormal changes, a third pain state, the abnormal chronic-pain-state can be triggered. Since that state does not exist during development, it is not setup to automatically return to the no-pain-state.

Luckily, through MBPC techniques, we can teach the nervous system how to reconnect with the normal no-pain-state and teach it how to unlearn the abnormal chronic-pain-state, over time. The system returns to the normal no-pain-state, with the ability to use the normal acute-pain-state for a new injury, followed again by the no-pain-state, as tissues heal.

Certain types of neurons, located in the spinal cord and some pain-related regions within the brain, are capable of neuroplasticity. As a form of learning, in response to changes in their environment, they are capable of altering their behaviors and of selecting different neurons in their environment to communicate with, thus reorganizing and forming new pathways. This includes initiating, learning, and establishing abnormal, chronic pain pathways, as well as, fortunately, re-establishing normal pain pathways.

We don't need to fear that once the nervous system creates abnormal, chronic pain patterns, we will have to suffer from chronic pain for forever. Regarding pain control, neuroplasticity is not limited to occurring only once, nor does it work in only one direction. CBi techniques direct neuroplasticity to help pain-related neurons unlearn abnormal and relearn normal, or nearly normal pain states, depending on the condition.

Since chronic pain is abnormal, complex conditions contributed to its creation. Once neuroplasticity resets normal pain pathways, perhaps the chances for chronic pain returning are low because the chance of those complex conditions recurring is low. Once normal pain processes are re-established for a particular condition and chronic pain is no longer an issue, a new condition may arise that brings chronic pain with it. Using CBi techniques again can help pain processing normalize again. The techniques can be applied over and over.

With chronic conditions that are acutely painful, pain control skills can help alleviate recurring acute pain, or help prevent abnormal chronic pain from taking hold. Following diagnosis and stabilization of chronic conditions that continually create new acute pain, applying pain control techniques can help the nervous system ignore that particular acute pain for reasonable periods of time. For continuous acute pain caused by a chronic condition to completely subside, depending on the condition and the individual's skill level, it can take only moments, or months, but it may take years.

For example, my 2004 right foot injury was a difficult case for re-establishing normal acute/no pain pathways. I applied chronic pain control skills from 2010 until 2014, when its chronic pain completely stopped. I was amazed that intrinsically controlling the pain could make it stop. Stopping continuous, acute pain from interstitial cystitis took a student a few months.

We intuitively knew that neuroplasticity occurred before technological advances made it possible to demonstrate it empirically in the neuroscience labs. Old dogs actually can be taught new tricks. For example, adults can learn how to play the piano by taking piano lessons and practicing diligently, intentionally changing their behaviors, thought patterns, and their mind.

In order for us to change from someone who cannot control pain into someone who can, CB Intrinsic chronic pain control techniques take advantage of neuroplasticity. When behaviors and thoughts change, the brain's flexible neural pathways can change, for the long-term, due to neuroplasticity. The CBi Touch and MBPC techniques utilize and actively nurture neuroplasticity, as often as needed, to re-establish and maintain normal pain states.

Neuroplasticity: Relearn to Reset.

Stress Sustains Pain

As mentioned earlier, acute pain does not cause harm, even though it hurts. Chronic pain is different. Regardless of whether or not actual tissue damage has been causally linked to the chronic pain condition by a doctor, all types of chronic pain indirectly lead to widespread tissue harm.

For example, chronic pain can induce chronic inflammation, by directly stimulating inflammatory cells. Inflammatory cells fight invader cells, but that part of the immune system is not sophisticated enough to distinguish our own cells from invader cells. Consequently, inflammation also damages our own cells. In that way, chronic pain causes harm by indirectly leading to inflammation.

Pain's perpetuation of long-term stress is another way that chronic pain causes harm, again indirectly. Long-term stress negatively impacts health by eventually causing illnesses involving organs, such as the kidneys, liver, and digestive tract, or by causing cardiovascular diseases, such as hypertension, and by reducing the quality of sleep or causing insomnia. Long-term stress even depresses the immune system, which will eventually lead to illness and disease. Chronic pain and long-term stress together conjure up quite a toxic brew.

Neurons in the pain pathways of our nervous system are closely associated with neurons related to emotions. They interact to modify each other along the way, as part of the interpretation process that takes place before pain is perceived. Stressful, negative emotions directly affect pain by making it worse, and in return, pain affects emotions negatively by making negative emotions worse.

The fact that negative emotions from long-term stress and chronic pain go hand-in-hand is one of the main reasons chronic pain is so unhealthy.

The unhealthy impacts of long-term stress not only harm us physically by increasing risks for illness and disease, but stress also impairs our ability to think clearly, which could, at times, make it more difficult to maintain relationships, resolve conflict effectively, exercise good judgment, act rationally, or remain focused to reach future goals. In so many ways, chronic pain, through long-term stress, reduces our quality of life, and changes who we are.

The instant we resist pain, we may notice a sudden tightening in the chest, due to the fight or flight response of stress. Stress immediately reinforces and amplifies pain symptoms. By earnestly trying to flee from pain, or by passionately fighting pain and feeling angry, stress levels substantially increase, which can substantially increase pain symptoms. Long-term stress and chronic pain feed off of each other and reinforce each other. They are directly proportional; if one increases, the other increases. It's a survival thing.

Increased stress can make pain seem more solid, more real, and more in control, as if pain were a tangible, real object. Survival instincts support stress and intensify pain perception, so we will give pain more weight, and have more incentive to take appropriate action to get help for the injury. For chronic pain, we need to get help primarily due to the ill effects of pain-related long-term stress. To reduce one, you must reduce both.

To reduce the occurrence, unpleasantness, and intensity of chronic pain, we must reduce automatic, instinctive tendencies toward creating more stress, no matter how justified we think stress is.

Pain-related stress seems justified because pain seems unfair, especially when it is chronic, and especially when it seems nothing can stop it. Getting angry feels rational, making it seem we have a right to get angry. The brain's comfort zone is to fixate on pain, get angry, and get stressed out about it. If not anger, then perhaps emotions like depression with isolation take over, but lying low does not reduce stress. It is a form of stress.

The emotions of stress are expressed by a wide range of behaviors, ranging from fight to flight to freeze. Anger is a form of fight. Depression, isolation, and fleeing are forms of flight. Fleeing from, getting angry about, or concentrating on the unfairness of chronic pain only serve to increase the stress, and thus, pain symptoms. We must flee from whatever causes an injury or resolve the illness or condition. Yet if we want to control chronic pain, we must control our instinctive tendency of getting stressed out about it, and intentionally do the opposite.

The brain discounts any intentions for actively reducing stress. It simply makes no sense to the brain to turn off stress when we feel pain. It's like trying to get water to run effortlessly up a steep cliff.

So, to control chronic pain, we have to ignore the brain's preferences. We literally have to take over the control and trick the brain.

To do the 'opposite', we don't merely try to feel 'positive' about pain to reduce the stress. Faking it until we make it does not work. We have several tricks, but for now, we reduce both stress and pain by changing perspective.

For example, to reduce pain's escalation of stress, we take advantage of the fact that pain is subjective. As mentioned earlier, pain and thoughts have a lot in common. They are both mind-stuff. They are part of our awareness, and we can control both through the same, our awareness. We approach pain from an intentional, objective, fact-based, non-instinctive perspective.

For another example, we must take measures to counteract futile urges to flee from the pain, or to feel overly fearful of it. We will change our perspectives about pain by intellectually separating the injury in the body from the actual perception of pain in the brain.

Perspective is a very powerful tool for redirecting and controlling mind-stuff. It may not sound hugely powerful, but since we can learn how to use the mind to shape the mind, our own mind, it actually is Powerful.

Emotion and Behavior

Subjective pain and stress hijack our thoughts. We can't think as clearly or creatively while fully absorbed in the pain and stress. Whether it is acute or chronic, pain causes us to slow down. We tend to put off getting things done. Serious pain causes us to stop whatever we were doing. Productivity on all levels tapers off. With chronic pain, the goals we once cared about may lose their meaning; they certainly lose their importance.

We may not be interested in doing the things we used to do before the injury or condition began. It's harder to feel interested in much of anything. We don't really want to invite people over or go to their houses. We may feel nauseous, have low energy, and feel depressed and frustrated. Since we hurt, we may become sedentary. We place the exercise routine on hold. We focus on pain as it becomes our main priority. Chronic pain can become a major component of who and what we think we are.

Pain even changes our sense of humor. We may not feel like laughing very much. We may feel less jovial about everything in general. Perhaps we become more cynical. Situations may seem unfair, and we may have feelings of anger more frequently. We will take things more personally. We may feel trapped by the pain. We feel we have lost control of life, and that our entire life, not just the exercise routine, is on hold. Chronic pain causes prolonged stress, and studies show that prolonged stress promotes chronic pain. It is a vicious cycle.

We know from science that prolonged or long-term stress leads to an increase in illness and disease, such as depression, irritable bowel syndrome, liver and kidney disease, osteoarthritis, diabetes, muscle wasting, hypertension, cancer and more, as mentioned earlier.

Controlling chronic pain through intrinsic methods helps decrease exposure to the ill effects of living with long-term stress. We must change the way we think about, process, and react to chronic pain. MBPC techniques change the overriding tendency to react into a more relaxed tendency to respond objectively to pain.

Thinking about pain objectively, while realizing that pain is subjective is essential for being able to respond to pain. It is helpful to understand how interactions between neurons, emotions, and stress affect chronic pain. Knowing how to change the way we react to pain is helpful, too. To learn how to convert reactivity into response, let's begin by reviewing how we typically react.

Typical reactions to pain:

- We often gasp and hold our breath or scream as we move away from what causes the pain (or grab where the pain originates, if from an organ or something inside).
- We may grimace, tighten our muscles, and pull in our arms or legs (becoming more compact as we tighten muscles to be better isolated away from the pain).
- Our stress levels instinctively increase.

- We want to do whatever it takes to make the pain stop.
- Any distinction between the tissue damage and the pain itself is absent.

Through our own personal experience, we also know that for each type of pain, for each person, and during each moment, our relationship with pain changes. We know there is a full range of discomfort, extending from mild, 'piece of cake to deal with' type of pain all the way to a very intense, overwhelming spinal cord pain that seems to reach out to the stars.

We may go through several stages while accepting our chronic pain condition. At first, we may approach it with disbelief. As it lingers, we deny and resist it. We fight it and feel angry. We fear it won't end, so we give up, stop fighting, repress, and try to suffer through it. Finally, if there are periodic breaks in the pain, we learn to put it in the back of our mind, somehow compartmentalizing it, so we can work and get on with life to the best of our ability. We trivialize it by rationalizing that other people might have it worse. We become resigned to our lack of control, and wish some new pill, or someone, or something else would control our pain and take it away.

Chronic pain can even consume the personality. Stress takes control and paints a dark picture for every situation. The unfairness of constant pain, the lack of quality of life, the unending suffering and contempt for the painful condition work together to reshape who we think we are. Being consumed by pain leaves little room for anything else. Who we used to be can become a distant memory.

Once we get to the final stages, whether pain is all consuming or it has been compartmentalized, we are so accustomed to dealing with it, in one way or another, that we can't remember what life was like before chronic pain began. We lose touch with who we really are.

It helps to remember that our perception of pain ultimately depends on which neural pathways are being used at a particular time. It's all about the neurons. Control the neurons and their pathways, and we can control pain. We are not stuck or lost forever.

Pharmaceuticals are designed to control specific pain neurons and their pathways. CB Intrinsic techniques control the same neurons and their pathways without requiring a pill or some outside resource, other than perhaps a caring friend, or the use of a clean feather duster to help us Touch places that are difficult to reach.

As with the Touch, MBPC techniques do not satisfy instinct or common sense or mind-stuff. They do not reinforce stress. They do not support, protect, amplify, or sustain pain. They do not result in the same response from pain that we feel when we react to pain. In fact, MBPC techniques result in an exact opposite response.

That makes sense because in order to go from being controlled by chronic pain all the way to controlling chronic pain, something within us has to change completely. We must mentally take a full 180 degree turn away from instincts to achieve the opposite of pain.

Ten Mindful Opposites

Don't be misled by the apparent simplicity of the following complex MBPC strategies. The effects are profound. Being able to unlearn chronic pain patterns depends on using these techniques. They help an adult's nervous system re-establish normal pathways for acute-pain followed by no-pain patterns, as tissues heal. Chronic pain patterns find it difficult to return.

Intense Visualization
Switch On Endorphin
Exercise May Ease Pain
Be Social – Don't Isolate
Relax Every Muscle Fiber
Reduce Anger and Anxiety
Take Conscious Deep Breaths
Smile and Laugh to Block Pain
Feel Enthusiastic and Lighthearted
Switch to Effective Perspective Thinking

1. Intense Visualization

We have all heard that we should be careful about what we wish for. We should also be careful about what we focus on. If pain is top-of-mind too often, those thoughts tend to strengthen pain because thinking about pain strengthens the neural pathways that support pain. Intensely visualizing away from pain is powerful, yet it needs to be applied skillfully to be effective.

Intensely focusing on anything other than pain can help reduce pain. Athletes and soldiers are less sensitive to pain, while they focus on their goal. Important projects with a deadline require a concentrated effort to remain focused. Pain, like extraneous thoughts, can be prevented from interfering with our full concentration and attention for the project. Focusing on a significant distraction can reduce pain by taking the mind's energy and attention away from the pain.

Have you noticed that when you focus on an engaging or all-consuming task, pain is forgotten for a while? Do you feel pain while you are asleep? No. But you can feel pain while dozing because dozing is not the same thing as being asleep. Sleep is the ultimate distraction.

Muscles are completely relaxed during restful sleep. By relaxing muscles, as much as they are during sleep, it is possible to temporarily prevent the perception of pain. Staying awake while simulating sleep, with nearly every muscle relaxed to the max is, oddly enough, exhausting. Unless we are actually sleeping, it is hard work to keep every single muscle completely relaxed at the same time.

Relaxing every muscle means that the impacts of stress are reduced, while the focus on relaxation is very intense. Concurrent pain is forgotten. Accomplishing that it is quite the challenge, though. Other distractions include surfing the net, reading a great book, watching a movie, or doing anything that truly interests you.

Attention doesn't have to be focused on something real. The first time I successfully stopped my severe trigeminal nerve pain for a few moments back in 1977,

I used visualization. Tricking the brain into stopping pain with visualization was most unexpected. The trick also relied on initiating the wave of comfort, peace, and joy that coursed through my entire body from head to toe. It included diverting 100% of my mind's focus toward anything other than the pain. Focus intensely and become one with something, anything other than pain. Let every aspect of that activity fill 100% of your senses. Intense visualization is extremely powerful.

If you are recovering from surgery, or if your condition is cyclical, intensely visualize or imagine how it will feel to be pain-free in six weeks or six months, or whenever you believe the pain will have had enough time to run its course or cycle to a stop. Now, don't just wish it. Literally reach into the future to feel the absence of your pain right now, if only for a moment. Make it real! Practice stretching that moment into minutes. This is an intense visualization worthy of full engagement.

Focusing on goals can take the mind away from pain but finding the right thing to focus on and having the right amount of focus need some preparation.

Suffering from chronic pain for a long time can make it difficult to remember the goals and engaging projects that used to matter. Focus and try to remember what mattered most. Remember what used to bring joy. Remember the needs that really counted. Select goals that could potentially engage every fiber of your being.

Figure out the needs or goals that would be easiest to accomplish right now. Plan how to accomplish them, but do not let the mind get stuck in its comfort zone of telling you to not even try. Strategize how to make them happen. Take a few days. Never let the brain tell you no. Memories about what used to matter will come back. Write them down. Make a list. Act as if pain is no longer the priority, even though your body tells you it still is.

All pain is a product of the brain, and only in that sense is it 'real'. Pain is different from a thought that comes in sentences. Pain is a perception made up of intensity, type, and location, along with the emotional and situational aspects that the brain attributes to it. Yet like a thought, the brain can be distracted away from it.

We can think of only one thing at a time. Once attention is taken completely away from pain, sometimes we can forget the pain for that time. Remaining focused intensely on something enjoyable is one proven way to prevent the mind from making too much pain. Do this with intention and conviction because the brain knows when you are faking it.

Some pain is so relentless, no amount of focusing will keep it at bay for more than a few moments at time. Cheat by also applying the Touch. Its effectiveness with MBPC will blow your mind, but that's okay.

Distractions work because the pain related regions of the brain are easily side-tracked. Pain can be forgotten periodically. As emotional stress and the situational aspects of the mind change, pain can become less unpleasant and more easily forgotten. Focus wholeheartedly on distractions. Focus on goals. Intensely focus on projects to lessen the intensity and emotional/situational aspects of the pain.

A pitfall of some distractions is that their effectiveness can end the moment we check back in with the pain because we wanted to make sure the distraction was working. Boom! The distraction is lost, and pain raises its ugly head again. Just like sleep, distraction effects last only as long as you are distracted.

One of the best ways to track success with distractions is to postpone checking-in. For example, notice that while fly-fishing all day last Saturday, there were times you were distracted enough that you did not feel pain. Remembering back is a safe way to gauge progress with distractions. Notice if pain seems to have occurred less often over the past two weeks; that type of thing. Remain immersed in the distractions; identify with those instead of identifying with pain. Think less about the pain without reflecting back, until much later to gauge your progress from a safe temporal distance.

Working on challenging physical goals can distract the mind from its perception of pain for quite a long time, or at least reduce it now and then, depending on the intensity, type of pain and condition. I realize this does not work for all types, or especially high levels of relentless pain, but distractions do reduce perceptions of most types of pain. Combined with the Touch, distractions can work much more effectively.

2. Switch On Endorphins

Our emotions are very fluid. Let's pretend you are waiting for an extremely positive and important phone call. Imagine how you feel every time the phone rings.

When it rings, your hopes go way up. You feel a rush of excitement coursing through your entire body. You become so excited! You answer the phone, but it is not who you had hoped. You feel disappointed. Later, the phone rings again. Your hopes shoot up and you are flying high because surely, they have had enough time to call you by now. You answer the phone, but it's a friend calling to ask if they can catch a ride with you in the morning. You are happy to hear from your friend, yet you are disappointed because it wasn't *the* call.

Excitement and disappointment continue to rise and fall every time the phone rings. No one else is in the room, and there is nothing pressing on your calendar. Your expectations and the phone are the only things affecting your mood. Can the 'phone' change your mood?

Because our brain/mind believes that how we feel depends on outside, extrinsic influences, it blames those extrinsic influences for everything bad that happens to us. It feels ecstatic when the phone rings because the ring sets off mind-made expectations – mental justifications for excitement. Finding a reason for excitement or disappointment, and determining how excited or disappointed to feel, is what minds do. The mind doesn't realize that the brain is solely responsible for all the neurons and biochemicals that literally 'create' how we feel, every time and always. The mind believes that something outside of us is the main reason for the emotions we experience. The mind is the last to realize how incorrect that is.

We realize the phone itself cannot force our emotions to change. We are not consciously trying to make our emotions change. It's the default setting of the mind. Mood depends on the brain/mind interpretation process, on which perspectives we choose to frame any situation, and we automatically follow wherever the mind leads. Continuing to blindly follow mind-made beliefs about what is real prevents us from moving forward with what is truly real about chronic pain control.

The mind never lets you realize that regardless of outside situations or reasons, regardless of your mood or attitude, the brain, with its biochemistry, is the sole reason for anything you feel, whether it is pain or emotion, or no pain.

It is good for us that the brain is the sole reason – the brain holds the solution, so control the brain. Instead of allowing the factory, default setting of the brain to control your mind on autopilot, be the pilot. Its biochemicals, the neurons with their interconnections, and many pain-related regions of the brain are all at our disposal. There are always choices. We are able to use the brain differently, at will, over and over again, without limit. This realization is powerful and it's critical for effectively mastering chronic pain control skills.

As soon as we learn how to become the pilot of the brain, to control our stress and emotions without needing an outside justification, like a phone call, being able to successfully control chronic pain is very near. It depends on being able to turn on pure enthusiasm or joy at any moment, regardless of the ruminations and objections of the mind. We must become our own change agent. Instead of expecting the mind to direct every single thing that defines us, we learn to instead consciously respond to our mind so we can redirect it to better suit our needs and preferences, striving toward molding healthier mind-sets for truly positive change.

To gain control of our pain pathways, begin the practice of less dependence or reliance on repetitious thoughts or false needs for justification. Forget that you think you need a really good reason, or 'a phone call' for feeling exuberant. Learn to feel a rush of enthusiasm whenever you want to, if for no other reason than it feels good, plus it's healthy. Toss out the mind's silly instinctive and misguided resistance and objections.

To learn how, first practice using imagination to turn the feelings of excitement and/or enthusiasm on for no apparent reason. It's not weird because we already do this without thinking about it, fairly often.

The difficult part of this practice is separating feelings of excitement from erroneous, conditional mind-made rules; detach the actual feelings of excitement from the conditions you only 'think' must be met so your mind would give you permission to feel excited. Start small.

Think back to remember something you felt excited and enthusiastic about. Visualize and focus on those moments to virtually relive them. Turn on and feel the same feelings now that you felt then. It's within you.

Or remember everything you can about your favorite vacation; the sights, smells, tastes, temperatures, the humidity, the sounds; remember everything. Practice allowing joy to turn on. Notice the inner workings of how it turns on. What happens first in your mind/body, then next and next? Memorize it to control and own it.

Practice your visualization, and take a slow, deep, conscious breath, in and out, as you relive and feel joy radiate. Do you feel the rush intensify throughout your body? Can you feel the inner peace, the exhilaration and bliss? Can you intensify those feelings even more? Can you make your whole body feel an ecstatic tingling sensation all-over, for no outside reason at all?

Notice everything about this rush. Memorize it. Learn how to recreate this rush of exuberance without using visualization. Turn on the rush as if you just flip a switch.

At first, feeling excitement without an outside reason may feel kind of wobbly or weird. It might seem harder than it was to ice or roller skate for the first time. If imagination isn't helping, do you have a favorite feel-good movie, or a favorite comedy? Watch it and practice turning on those feel-good feelings at will, on purpose.

Culture has us convinced that we need an outside reason for feeling ecstatic, but that is incorrect. Having a good inside reason works equally well. Improving health is the best inside reason. The fact that this rush is healthy is the reason. It leads to stopping chronic pain, and that alone leads to feelings of outrageous empowerment. Don't worry; wobbly and weird will disappear.

Once you learn how to feel excited for no reason (other than you have decided to feel excited), practice switching that on in a flash. Don't test the waters to ease into it. Make it happen in a flash – turn on the switch. Make your whole body instantly zing with exuberance!

If your condition allows, while breathing deeply, add a genuine smile and let yourself laugh! Feel the tingling wave as it rushes up and down, and all around your body. This is how we are meant to experience life.

To use stress as our comfort zone is the nonsensical, unhealthy opposite; why would we want to waste so much time and energy, every single day, every waking hour creating stress?

Instead, practice this healthy rush of enthusiasm every chance you get, even when you aren't feeling pain. No one is watching. Just do it. Your entire body, mind and spirit will thank you.

Let's understand this at a deeper level. This rush of excitement is the fastest and easiest way to lessen stress significantly enough to reduce pain. Once you discover the truth of this for yourself, diminishing pain is more than a good enough reason to feel ecstatic and enthusiastic at will.

Performing this 'rush' is Universally Healthy for the entire body. And unlike mimicking sleep, this technique does not require very much energy to reduce pain. In fact, this releases a boost in energy.

As you smile, while feeling the rush, remember to release tension, too. Relax. Let joy replace the stress and tension. Practicing this is very healthy for the immune system, organ maintenance, blood pressure, memory, digestion, the libido, relationships, and the well-being of your entire mind, body, and spirit!

When someone is stressed, everyone in the room can feel their stress. Calm, peace, and enthusiasm are just as contagious as stress, but unlike stress, they are healthy. When you practice this in the presence of others, they can feel your joy as it permeates the room, and they can see the calm confidence in your face. They will want to practice this, too. The rush creates a naturally healthy and very safe high, which has practically no limits nor any negative side effects. That's a skill worth practicing.

As the topic of this section implies, this is all about turning on 'endorphin' to stop pain. Our bodies produce natural painkillers called opiates. By turning the rush on naturally, we purposefully turn on the neurons which release these painkilling, endorphin-like opiates.

Back in the 1970's, scientists first discovered our natural opiates - enkephalin, endorphin and dynorphin. There is a story behind how endorphin got its name.

When morphine controls pain, it chemically mimics our 'endogenous' opiates and tricks our body into using it to kill pain. Endogenous refers to biochemicals that are made naturally by the body, for the body. When scientists discovered the specific endogenous molecule that morphine mimics, they named it by combining the two words '*endo*genous' and 'mo*rphine*' to get **endorphin.** Pharmaceuticals kill pain. Endorphins kill pain. One kind is extrinsic, and the other kind is intrinsic. Guess which is actually healthy.

(By convention, 'opioid' refers to all opiates, whether they are synthetic drugs, opium based or endogenous. For endogenous opioids, I use the words endorphin for endorphin specifically, and 'endorphins' plural to include all endogenous opioids. Endorphin(s)-releasing neurons are located throughout the nervous system.)

We switch on natural endorphin-releasing neurons and their pathways through our chosen state of mind. Since it only takes a couple of seconds, we can do it at any time. It is a pleasurable way to trick the brain into stopping chronic pain. This changes lives for the better. Turning on endorphins is essential and is the crux of the matter for all CB Intrinsic Chronic Pain Control techniques because *endorphins turn off stress and pain*.

Stimulating endorphin neurons within the brain results in excited, joyful, ecstatic, and even euphoric feelings because endorphin pathways turn on the brain's pleasure centers. Pain control is all about the neurons.

We are even able to consciously turn on endorphin on through a back door; smiling or laughing also leads to feeling excited or ecstatic. Endorphin-releasing neurons are directly turned on in the brain by the smile-creating muscles of the face. Once turned on, the endorphin-releasing neurons turn on the brain's pleasure center neurons. The brain cannot tell which way it is going; the smile can come first, or the reason can come first. Only the mind notices, and we control the mind.

This is why it is important to keep the mind's objections from interfering with this process; its typical insistence on first having a solid reason for feeling excited or joyful does not take into account our ability to directly turn on endorphin with a smile. Practice triggering this excited, enthusiastic, endorphin painkilling rush without needing reasons, imagination, or thoughts. You can turn endorphin on just as you can swallow whenever you want to, with or without food.

Once you are practiced at stopping chronic pain, due to mindfully turning on endorphin (that morphine mimics, hence it kills pain), your mind will finally learn it has more than enough high-quality reasons for welcoming this change.

Then it becomes easier. We might even say it is like running a blast of water down a sandy hill; the rut deepens quickly, and the effects spread far and wide. Learning to turn on endorphins is not a steep learning curve because successfully learning how feels so good. That's nature's way of telling us this is healthy and right.

It is not necessary for you to understand how neurons use endorphins to stop chronic pain or to know where endorphins work within the nervous system for this to be effective. Just know that research gives this a sound scientific basis.

Endogenous opioids are our body's own natural, internal, intrinsic painkillers, and we can turn them on as if we flipped a switch. They occur only in natural levels, so they do not disrupt our natural balance, our body's homeostasis. Quite the opposite. Turning them on is healthy. It just takes practice. Be the pilot.

Thinking back, Intense Visualization and Switch On Endorphins are the techniques I first unwittingly used in 1977 to stop my parotid gland's intense trigeminal nerve pain. It is possible to visualize and focus on something (even if it is imaginary) so intensely that it becomes (subjectively) real. And I noticed, not knowing I was switching on endorphins, the rush that stopped intense trigeminal nerve pain for a few precious moments. It worked from the 'top-down', from my head to my toes, and from fingertips to fingertips. Stopping pain intrinsically saved my life.

Acute pain is felt, but having mastered it by now, my mind instantly feels no chronic pain as it automatically turns on endorphins without needing visualizations or thoughts. My skill is no longer limited to moments of pain relief. Endorphins run silently, automatically in the background, helping prevent the return of chronic pain. Switching on endorphins is healthy for the immune system and is powerful against both stress and pain.

3. Exercise May Ease Pain

Mild to strenuous exercise, based on your abilities (BOYA) and when the illness or condition allows, is our next strategy. Exercise can lift spirits. Given enough time, exercising can stimulate endorphin pathway. Pain is subjective and exercise can change its landscape.

Exercise helps clear the body of medications and toxins. Drink lots of water while exercising to help the liver and kidneys process those chemicals. Exercise increases energy reserves. Exercise increases heart rate and strengthens heart muscle. It seems that exercising would cause fatigue, however the more you exercise, the more your muscles get into shape. Strong muscles burn more fuel because muscle fibers burn blood sugar, simply because it is around. The body feels more energized.

Exercising improves overall health. The mechanical motion of skeletal muscles helps move blood through veins more efficiently. Lymph vessels of the immune system track alongside arteries (except in the brain). A faster pumping heart pushes blood through the arteries more quickly. Faster artery pumping action massages lymph vessels more vigorously, which may help move lymph and immune cells through the lymph system more effectively. The lymph system has many roles. For our purposes, it is where many immune cells hang out, while checking the lymph fluid for foreign invaders, such as bacteria or viruses that have entered the blood.

With the lymph fluid moving faster throughout the body, immune cells travel throughout the body more efficiently and effectively in their search for foreign invaders, and even cancerous cells.

Exercise also relieves stiffness and improves muscle tone. Reducing stiffness reduces pain. Scar tissue or connective tissue adhesions are a common source of painful sensations. Exercise and stretching can help tear away and breakup adhesions (laugh through the temporary pain, if you are able), which leads to fewer reasons for pain down the road. Stronger muscles and better muscle tone can promote healthier and more stable joints, which may suffer less future injury and pain.

Suggestions for exercise (BOYA) include swimming, cycling with an elliptical, walking, singing, dancing, vacuuming, reaching for things high and low, and resistance training.

4. Be Social – Don't Isolate

We are social beings. Don't be a hermit. Supportive friends can help reduce chronic pain. Exercise with friends. Go for walks with friends. Work out with your new friends from the gym. Get involved in sports again, if practical. Combine exercise and laughter with friends. Practice switching on endorphins together for no good reason! Enjoy yourself.

Do you remember when we listed examples for how pain changes our daily lives? We talked about not having fun or feeling like laughing. We talked about not wanting to do anything, preferring to just lay low, not wanting to go over to friends' houses, or having them over as often. We sit at home in pain. The pain controls us. Pain can become all we think about. We talk about pain in Online groups. We reinforce and strengthen each other's pain. We stress out about it together. Pain sometimes becomes who 'we' are, in some pain groups.

Has it become who you are? Which one came first, the stress or the pain? Try to clearly remember what your personality was like before pain took it over.

Instead of becoming a hermit in pain, leave the house to get exercise and stimulate the mind. Finding something to do with friends could prevent the mind from constantly thinking about or identifying with pain. Ask people over and likewise, accept invitations to go to their houses. Pamper yourself. Do whatever brings joy, inner peace, and tranquility. Soak in the hot tub, spend a day at the spa, or spend time in your favorite sanctuary, such as the mountains, beside a beautiful river, the beach, or visualize your favorite vacation.

Lose yourself in what used to relax you and what used to matter to you. Have lots of fun. Encourage conversations and activities with friends in order to direct the brain away from identifying with pain. Be careful and observant – try to not allow the topic of your pain to hijack these new conversations.

If you lack something interesting to talk about, because pain has occupied your thoughts for so long, listen to your friends' stories. Develop new interests through them. It takes time to rediscover who you used to be, and who you truly are. Pain is not who you are.

5. Relax Every Muscle Fiber

Pain tenses muscles and won't let the them go. So, another opposite that releases pain is to intentionally and deeply relax all muscles. Muscles are relaxed during sleep, which partly explains how sleep combats pain. The goal is to reach a sleeping state for every muscle fiber. The results from purposefully relaxing every muscle fiber, as much as is humanly possible while remaining awake, can be more effective against pain than sleeping.

Set aside perhaps an hour for practicing this awakened state of sleep, ensuring beforehand that nothing will distract or interrupt you. Focus on maintaining total muscle relaxation. No muscle should feel any tension. If part of a muscle feels tense, relax it more. Let the entire body go limp and keep it there. Allow your muscles to remain asleep, while your mind remains wide awake.

To support the body during this total relaxation, sit in a chair with a headrest and ottoman, use a recliner, or practice this reclined on a bed. Focus entirely on keeping each muscle completely, 100% relaxed. While attempting to achieve this level of nearly zero tension, the mind must remain 100% focused as the muscles themselves fall deeply asleep.

Continue scanning your body to relax any muscles that have returned to increased tension levels. Remember to actively focus on full-body muscle relaxation – nothing else. There won't be room for pain in the brain during this sustained concentration on muscle relaxation.

Practice releasing tension from the muscle fibers more and more completely each moment, more deeply than you think possible, while remaining fully awake.

Pain may return the moment tension returns to any muscle, regardless of where that muscle is located in relation to the pain. Don't stress. Put the muscles to sleep. Locate the tense muscle to relax it instantly, while keeping all other muscular and emotional tensions at bay. Notice how quickly pain disappears without a trace.

This requires a lot of energy because continuous and highly focused concentration, unlike sleep, requires a tremendous amount of energy. The rewards include bliss, exhilaration and stopping pain - basically any pain. Pain may not return if relaxation is maintained long and often enough. As with everything else, the more this is practiced, the more effective it becomes. Aim for sustaining five minutes of pain-free 'zero tension' at first, with a goal of eventually sustaining it for 30 minutes.

Admittedly, this Relax Every Muscle Fiber technique is very challenging, but it is rewarding in equal measure, and is worthy of Congratulations for Success.

6. Reduce Anger and Anxiety

The deeply ingrained, default or reactive factory settings of the brain naturally prioritize perceiving and amplifying pain. They act quickly, like water flowing down a steep hill in its deeply eroded rut because default settings are instinctive.

The nervous system is rigged so that the more you feel pain, the less you feel joy. It makes sense that negativity increases stress, and that stress beneficially increases pain because feeling pain is vital for personal safety. The default settings of the mind naturally lean toward negativity, if only to enhance the perception of physical pain. Reactivity increases stress and increases pain.

By reacting to injury, our bodies increase stress and pain, just as surely as water reacts to gravity and runs downhill. Stress covers a full range, from rage and anger to irritation, and from anxiety and frustration down to avoidance and freezing up. All are stressful behaviors and signs of stress. Anger and fear increase pain. Anticipating that something will be very painful increases anxiety levels, and those increase pain. Negative moods increase pain. While angry, pain becomes worse. The opposites are also true.

We are stuck in that rut with stress and pain until we become observant, watch what the mind is doing, effectively intervene when pain is unnecessary, change the natural flow and learn to respond rather than react.

Responding is the opposite of reacting, and a skill learned through mindfulness-based techniques. To reduce stress and pain, we teach the mind to respond rather than react to pain. While feeling less angry, sensations of pain feel less unpleasant. Enthusiasm and relaxation decrease pain. A truly positive mood correlates inversely with pain intensity; the more you feel joy, the less you feel pain (joy $\leftrightarrow$ endorphins = our natural painkillers).

Within the nerves, spinal cord, brainstem, and brain, emotion and pain modify each other. The negative emotions of stress increase pain, and pain increases stress, which in turn increases the unpleasantness and intensity of pain. The interactions run back and forth.

The **More Stress Equation** demonstrates how fight or flight, anger or fear increase when we can't stop, predict, or control pain. This applies to stress about a neighbor's barking dog as much as it applies to perceptions of pain.

More Stress Equation:

$$\begin{array}{r} \textbf{Can't Stop It} \\ + \textbf{Can't Predict It} \\ \underline{+ \textbf{Can't Control It}} \end{array}$$

More Stress

Because their effects are cumulative, each component contributes to the other for increasing the negative impacts of stress. Whenever any or all three terms of the **More Stress Equation** worsen, stress will rise.

Pain shares this equation with stress, since they have a positive relationship; they rise and fall together.

For example, I feel angry because I am in pain now, and I can't stop it. I'm angry because I'm afraid it won't ever stop. When pain does stop, I'm afraid it will return. I'm angry that I can't make plans because I can't predict when pain will leave or when it will return. I'm afraid of the pain because I can't control it.

Anger and anxiety feed on each other; each validates the other. Each adds to and increases the impact of the other. They affect all of our emotions. The negative emotions naturally bleed into and negatively affect our quality of life. Stress is contagious, so the negative emotions adversely affect the moods and quality of life of other people in the room.

This process easily perpetuates without any work or extra energy because this is instinctive. Stress is the default setting of the brain, and thus the mind.

We are so accustomed to stress that it controls our reactions more than we can realize. It's a constant state of mind, running unobserved in the background. We don't think we are stressed because the mind needs to compare and contrast in order to notice something. The constancy of stress prevents us from comparing and contrasting, so although it is in plain sight, stress hides from our awareness. Regardless of how complex and confusing this may seem, the bottom line is, we are usually stressed. We are primed to feel pain.

144

We can illustrate how stress and pain feed off of each other with a **Stress/Pain Positive-Feedback Loop.**

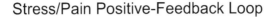

Stress/Pain Positive-Feedback Loop

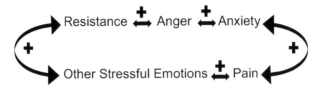

Leads to:
Increased Unpleasantness
Increased Pain Intensity
Increased Pain Frequency
Increased Pain Duration

The feedback is considered 'positive' because each component enhances the results of the other. Enhancing stress and pain leads us further away from what used to be normal. It is a loop because each spurs the others on, in all directions. The loop will continue until we use special tools to interupt and intervene.

We set ourselves up for worse pain by increasing stress and negative emotions of the loop. The primary components of pain, the unpleasantness of it, and its intensity are increased significantly in that way. Feeding the loop also increases the frequency of pain, so pain is felt more often, more times during the day, and more days out of the month. Of course, when increased intensity and frequency are involved, there is also the chance of increased duration.

Increasing stress and pain in this positive-feedback loop can increase pain's duration on multiple levels. It may last for a longer period of time each time it hurts, and it may hurt for a longer period of time overall, stretching out into the future, for perhaps years.

Therefore, as it is with typical reactions from feeling pain, we need do the opposites. We must reverse the **More Stress Equation** and the positive signs in the Loop must become negative to end this loop.

Thinking about a similar situation, we do not get stressed out about an itch in the same way we stress out about pain. That is because we can usually control an itch by scratching it. Since we can control most itches, we aren't afraid that an itch won't stop. We are not concerned about being unable to predict when or if it will return, because we easily control most itches again by merely scratching it again to stop it again.

Let's apply that to pain. For the **More Stress Equation**, 'Can't Control It' is the most essential component for turning this all around. To reverse the most important term in the equation, we make it so we 'Can Control It'. All of the rest will fall into place.

Utilizing any of the CB Intrinsic techniques successfully to control pain, the **More Stress Equation** reverses into its opposite, the **Less Stress Equation**.

Less Stress Equation:

CAN Stop It
+ ~~Can't Predict It~~   (cancels out)
+ CAN Control It

Less Stress

Notice that with the ability to control pain, two terms (not just one) are reversed into their opposites. Once we 'CAN Control It', we 'CAN Stop It'. Of the three terms, only 'Can't Predict It' remains. That is not a concern with pain for the same reason it is not a concern with an itch. 'Can't Predict It' abruptly drops out of the equation.

Applying opposites for the Loop, if we decrease (↓) typical forms of stressful emotions using MBPC, we decrease (↓) pain, which reverses the Loop's effects, resulting in less, rather than more stress and pain.

Stress/Pain Negative-Feedback Loop

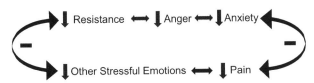

Leads to:
　　Decreased Unpleasantness
　　Decreased Pain Intensity
　　Decreased Pain Frequency
　　Decreased Pain Duration

Reducing Stress Reduces Pain

We know that decreasing or stopping pain will instantly decrease negative stress levels. It is also true that decreasing resistance to pain, feelings of anger and anxiety, plus decreasing other negative stressful emotions will decrease pain. If we reverse the loop into a Negative-Feedback Loop, it will have a normalizing effect. Stress and pain are still positively correlated; rather than enhancing how much they increase together, now they enhance how much they decrease together.

Less pain leads to feeling better, which leads to less stress, obviously, but less stress also leads to less pain. Less resistance, less fighting against pain by accepting that there is pain reduces anger and anxiety, while other stressful emotions are reduced, too. This positive correlation serves to likewise reduce all of the components of pain. It too is a loop, so it reduces stress and pain even more. Negative feedback helps the body normalize.

MBPC techniques effectively reduce or stop pain by negatively impacting stress. The negative emotional components of pain diminish, so the unpleasantness of pain decreases, and stress decreases further. The perception of pain becomes less overwhelming, and its intensity, frequency, and duration decrease, while stress decreases even more. Turning on endorphin takes care of the rest. Endorphin easily turns off residual stress. Endorphin won't let you feel Anger and Joy at the same time. Joy Wins. Over time, normal pain pathways can be re-established. This is powerful stuff.

Once we have control, we can stop worrying about pain so much. That is not to say we give up or that we no longer care about pain. This is not about putting up and 'dealing with it'. Instead, we have the upper hand! Pain no longer has the upper hand. It has lost its power. We have the Power! And having any degree of control over pain is a powerful weapon against stress, too.

What will replace all the time we could have spent experiencing chronic pain, anger, anxiety, fear, and other negative emotions? Their opposites replace them, of course. We feel empowered and are less of a victim to chronic pain. Pain directs and defines lifestyle less often, so quality of life improves. Instead of pain, we feel joy more often. We rediscover who we were meant to be!

7. Take Conscious Deep Breaths

(If your condition allows you to breathe deeply without causing harm (BOYA), imagine this scenario):

Suddenly, jolts of pain begin screaming at you. Muscles tighten and pull you in, making you smaller as you tense up and cower to the pain. You are compressed. With extreme pain, it is hard to expand and fill your lungs. The ribs want to stay constricted and tight, as if the body can't remember how to breathe. Instead, force yourself to take a deep breath and breathe!

You may find, as I have, that it takes effort to breathe through intense pain in the back, hip, leg, arm, etc. Count to three and force yourself to breathe in deeply!

Something that silences pain very effectively, through tricking the mind, is to take a slow, deep, conscious breath, or take several of them. For a conscious breath, we focus on every single aspect of the breath, while we intentionally breathe through the pain. If you immerse yourself in noticing every part of the breath, you are conscious of it, which makes pain more difficult to hold onto. This is an interesting phenomenon.

To practice, enjoy a relaxed, conscious, deep breath by focusing on the fresh air entering through your nose and/or mouth. Feel it as the cooler air fills your throat and air passages. Feel your ribs as they and your lungs expand. Imagine your blood carrying fresh oxygen from your lungs to all of the cells of your body. During your exhale, visualize carbon dioxide leaving the blood in your lungs to exit your body and mix with the outside air. Notice and feel the skin and every muscle in your body. Feel how alive your tissues are. Feel how the skin of your fingers and toes tingles.

It's amazing how well a conscious breath works to evaporate pain. Often, screaming pain evaporates as we force our ribs to expand for a deep, conscious breath, while focusing on every aspect of that breath.

Try conscious, deep breathing to control intense pain. It works with almost any pain, but the stark contrast is more obvious when an intense pain suddenly stops. It seems to go "poof". Breathe again to fight back the pain, pause, and take a conscious breath again. Include laughter, too. This works well during physical therapy.

Endorphins are found in the brain and throughout the body. Turn endorphins and their painkilling pathways ON throughout your brain and body, as much as possible, by including a smile with conscious, deep breathing. Feel the wave, the rush of comfort, as it floods the body. Feel the surge of pleasure, joy, and bliss. If feelings are difficult for you to detect, perhaps you will recognize them at first by a tingling sensation in the back of your neck.

8. Smile and Laugh to Dissolve Pain

Whenever we feel happy or have happy thoughts, we smile. We all know that smiling is contagious. When we watch someone that is smiling or laughing, we smile or laugh, too, and feel happy with them.

There is a third smile scenario, and we mention it yet again because it is so important. Unless a condition or injury makes it painful to smile or laugh (we do not want to cause further harm), by merely contracting the smile muscles of the face to form a genuine smile, we will feel happier. Brains don't care if the physical smile itself or a reason for being happy came first. Only a mind cares which happens first because the mind wants a reason first, or it will make it feel silly to smile. Yet whether we smile because we had a happy thought first, catch a contagious smile, or 'force' a genuine smile onto our face without a reason, the brain will make us feel happy. Minds are stubborn, while brains are easily tricked.

As it is with feeling enthusiastic or excited for no reason except to turn on endorphins for their healing effects, the important point about this is *using muscles that form a genuine smile directly turn endorphin on in the brain.* Those endorphin pathways activate chain reactions that even travel down the spine to stop pain.

The more you utilize pain control, endorphins, the pleasure center, and pain control pathways, the stronger they become. The stronger they are, the more effectively we control chronic pain, and the sooner those pathways become our second nature, our preferred new normal.

Stress generating pathways weaken when we use them less often. To help avoid using stress pathways, think about them less often. Thinking about them less often does not include concentrating on 'think about them less often'. Concentrating on 'stopping stress' only serves to strengthen stress, because thinking about stress, for any reason, reinforces and strengthens it.

That makes sense once we realize the brain does not distinguish 'thinking about trying not to be stressed' from actually being stressed. Focusing on and thinking about 'reducing the negatives in life' cause us to focus almost exclusively on the negatives in life, in order to avoid them. That only reinforces our negativity. We become more stressed by thinking about stress and stressing over the fact that we are still stressed. It can become an endless, viscous, lifelong, stressed-out cycle.

To weaken stress, replace it with smiles and laughter (BOYA). Concentrate on the smiles and laughter. Thinking about and practicing smiles and laughter will effortlessly strengthen the stress-fighting endorphin pathways, while it inadvertently, without thinking about it, weakens stress pathways, due to their lack of use.

Turning on endorphins by creating a smile applies to a full-face or nearly full-face smile. Such a smile engages the lips, cheeks, and eyes. I call it a genuine smile, regardless of whether or not we start out with a reason first.

Smirks are similar to smiles because smirks cause the lips to turn upward, but the brain knows a smirk is not a smile. Some of the signals between the facial muscles and the brain are missing, so smirks don't work.

Genuine smiles, on the other hand, have all of the necessary muscle/neuron connections that lead to turning on all of the areas of the brain that lead to activating endorphins globally, as an entire, whole-body experience. We are so lucky! Feel free to indulge.

As with genuine smiles, laughter works really well, too. Laughter is even used by the brain as an instinctive antidote to lower extreme stress levels.

Have you noticed that sometimes laughter happens at the most inappropriate times? When we are mortified or over-the-top remorseful, when stress levels are higher than we can stand, we might start laughing uncontrollably. Here the mind uses laughter as a defense mechanism or a strategy to reduce very high stress levels. It's automatic and we can't help it. Luckily, laughter works equally well to reduce intense chronic pain, in two stages.

First, laughter reduces the intense 'unpleasantness' that accompanies severe pain, thus making it more bearable. Secondly, quieting brain regions that are responsible for the emotional, unpleasant qualities of pain indirectly contributes to stopping pain by engaging more pain-stopping pathways that stretch from the brain down through the spinal cord; Top-Down pain control.

Stress supports chronic pain, but laughter does not. We need, and now know how to flip our instincts and extrinsic mind-beliefs around, in exchange for intrinsic, direct-brain connected solutions, because when someone laughs, they actually do have something to be happy about - they suffer less stress and less pain.

Smiles and laughter directly turn endorphin on in the brain, which turns on the pleasure centers, which tone down negative emotions. Endorphins in the body stop pain, just as morphine does. Reducing stress reduces negative emotions, which reduces the unpleasantness of pain, so pain becomes more bearable. Smiles and laughter lift spirits. Feel the wave of comfort as endorphins rush through your body, from head to toe, from fingertips to fingertips, tickling the back of your neck.

9. Feel Enthusiastic and Lighthearted

Remembering to feel enthusiasm or to find a positive perspective helps me reduce fears of new pain control 'opportunities' when they arise. In a way, stopping pain is something to look forward to because controlling it turns on the pleasure centers. (That makes sense because endorphins, from the Top-Down, directly turn on pleasure centers in the brain.) And, I can use it to help you. Do you remember that in the Journey section I mentioned feeling positive about painful challenges to

154

use as opportunities to learn more to help my students? Genuine positivity contributes positively for pain control.

Since pleasure is a natural by-product of practicing MBPC techniques for pain control, another episode with pain immediately becomes another reminder to feel enthusiastic. This paradigm shift is very healthy.

Controlling pain enthusiastically directly results in lightheartedness, which is another skill that grows stronger with endorphin use over time. Enthusiasm and lightheartedness become the brain's new normal.

Trying to be enthusiastic doesn't work (like a smirk), but being enthusiastic is very effective. Since faking is a type of resistance toward whatever is, which is stress in disguise, it makes sense that faking enthusiasm is an oxymoron, and results in the opposite of what we want.

Enthusiasm cannot be faked. Fake it until you make it doesn't apply. Enthusiasm is a direct result of turning on enough endorphin to kill stress, and is the basis of your new, altered reality. These techniques realign and redesign what is now 'real' within your mind-made world.

Looking up antonyms and synonyms for enthusiasm is an interesting exercise. Reading the list of antonyms is fairly depressing, so I will spend zero time there; but you can look into it.

Selecting from the list of synonyms for the words that reflect the intentions of this work, I would select zeal, joy and joyfulness, eagerness, energy, spirit, interest, earnestness, exhilaration (what I feel as pain stops), life (what I get to experience more fully once pain is gone), vivacity, and zest. I would add intention, because enthusiasm and intention are positively correlated and intertwined; when one goes up, so does the other.

Enthusiasm is a natural by-product of first switching endorphin on from inside the brain, and it enriches the entire body. Enthusiasm enriches all experiences. This way the term 'positive' takes on an entirely new meaning.

Enthusiasm is not a false positive because there are no judgments focused on identifying negatives that should be avoided nor beliefs that avoidance of negatives leads to positivity. Judgments only lead to false positives.

Enthusiasm is not about judging good or bad, positive, or negative. Enthusiasm is a 'true positive'. It is a positive within which negativity does not coexist. It celebrates inclusiveness. It values all. Enthusiasm is not a range, and it changes only in intensity. Its waters run deep, and then deeper still. Euphoria follows enthusiasm in degree. Both are very healthy for mind/body/spirit. An inadvertent by-product of using MBPC techniques is that they help us access a sense of Grace, which effortlessly softens chronic pain with its blanket of calm.

Lightheartedness is the opposite of being in a state of stress. As with stress, others can sense your lighthearted nature. They may not recognize that state of mind for what it is, but they like it. Fortunately for others, it is as contagious as stress. Lightheartedness can fill a room. The smiles lightheartedness generates may help reduce everyone's stress, soften everyone's mood, and dissolve everyone's perceptions of emotional and physical pain by turning endorphins on throughout their whole body.

Looking at synonyms for lighthearted that fit in this context, I would choose the following:

- *Buoyant* - because having faith that pain control will handle any challenge brings joy to lift us up,
- *Bright and cheerful* - because once the master level is reached, the gray skies of chronic pain potentially remain forever lifted,
- *Playful* - because controlling pain is fun,
- *Upbeat* - because you can stop unnecessary pain right away, or reduce it significantly right away, and then potentially stop it completely,
- *Resilient* - because whenever I experience severe chronic pain, I know it is possible to regain control and stop it by applying CB Intrinsic Touch and MBPC techniques together.

Endorphin and pleasure centers of the brain, plus other pain reducing pathways employed by the MBPC Top-Down techniques, bring on lightheartedness and peace of mind. With euphoria and enthusiasm in full force, pain fades away.

Lightheartedness and enthusiasm pour out of us. Switching on all of the endorphin types of neurons in the brain and body helps achieve full-body relaxation. By adding a deep breath/smile at the same time, further relaxation reduces stress and pain. MBPC skills help make all situations more exciting, rewarding and productive, while they reduce perceptions of pain.

Of course, we return to the stressed-out state of mind any split second that the brain/mind choses to go back into its rut. Try to not worry or create negative emotions about that fact. It's OK. It reminds us to practice our MBPC skills. The rewards of less stress, less pain, thus better health are easy to achieve, and worth the effort.

Through neuroplasticity, becoming enthusiastic and lighthearted will become your new comfort zone, the new default setting, the brain's favorite new rut. The stubborn mind may even whisper a thank you, eventually.

10. Use Effective Perspective Thinking

This is all about paradigm shifting to redirect perspectives to their opposites for more effective mind-sets. Let's go back in time to about 20 years before I figured out how to control pain. This was my 23rd surgery. I had apparently reached my psychological limit and could no longer accept having to wake up in so much pain following surgery. While nurses were wheeling me down the hall on a gurney, toward the operating room for a dreaded surgery, I suddenly felt like a helpless test subject or lab rat and spiraled into a full-blown panic attack. I had no control over myself, my bad luck, or the surgery. I believe I panicked because I feared waking up, post-surgery in a heap of pain, since I had always woken up in a heap of pain from surgeries in the past.

Whatever the cause for that panic attack was, it was a valuable and significant turning point for me. I vowed to never have a panic attack ever again. I believe this is when the notion of finding and working with opposite responses began developing for me.

My very first conscious 'opposite' was that I would not have a panic attack ever again. How could I ensure it wouldn't happen? I decided to not have any more surgeries, period. However, that was not well thought out. And as it turned out, that 'opposite' couldn't hold water because surgeries continued. The trick was or is to figure out the most rational and effective opposites.

Learning how to discover the most effective opposite changed my outlook on how to best move forward regarding most things in life from then on. Our minds are biased toward stress; we are born that way. We need to do the most effective opposite that will unravel prolonged stress, and allow us to make better choices, with patience and a clearer mind.

For my 24th surgery and not knowing if this related opposite would be effective, I asked the nurses and doctors for permission to walk myself into the operating room, instead of being wheeled in on a lab rat's gurney. The wonderful team decided to let me try it. Walking-in and climbing onto the operating table, to position myself for the surgery, made me feel like a member of the team. I didn't feel like a victim. I felt empowered. That was the right opposite, and I have had no more panic attacks before going into surgery.

The mechanics of changing from victim to team member stopped triggering uncontrollable, negative emotions related to pain. I was afraid the pain following surgery would be unbearable. The brain/mind matches thoughts to emotions, without needing anything in real-time to support it. I was not yet suffering from the pain, but my mind was certain I would, so in a way, I was already suffering from the pain. That imagined suffering equaled 'reality' for my mind's internal world.

On the other hand, looking at the situation of preparing for surgery from a team member's perspective, fear of pain was not the issue. Preparing for a successful surgery was the issue. The team had a task to perform, and I played my part in ensuring its success. My brain gave me positive emotions to match my team member thoughts aimed toward positive success. Employing the subjectivity of pain, plus positive emotions from the team member perspective have effectively helped me either reduce or erase fear and stress about potential surgery pain, ever since. This also requires intentional focus, and fewer distractions or contagious negative emotions from other people immediately preceding the surgery.

Employing an opposite thought or behavior is an example of a paradigm shift. Paradigm shifts are dramatic, and they are necessary for helping the mind change from a lesser perspective to a more effective perspective. Use paradigm shifts as often as you can for creating balance, realigning, and redesigning your mind's new reality of your internal world.

Critical thinking is required to figure out the effective perspective for the paradigm shift. 'Critical' is not about being cynical. It's about looking beyond the mind's current beliefs and analyzing paradigm shifts. Critical thinking requires us to pause, step back, prioritize getting to the root of the issues, analytically discover more facts, release old, invalid beliefs, and consider the most effective options. Critical thinking implies embracing new facts to view reality from a better perspective. Investigate the most effective perspectives to discover the most effective opposites for each situation.

Let's apply critical thinking and paradigm shifting to controlling chronic pain. We begin with chronic pain controlling us, yet we'd like to turn that around so we can control chronic pain instead. Those Are Opposites.

Let's look closely at the situation. When the body reacts to a painful stimulus from tissue damage, the brain instinctively does whatever it can to support and amplify that pain. It enhances pain so you will fight it. The body's reactions to pain guarantee increasing stress to will make you feel pain more intensely, so it will seem more solid, which 'helps ensure you'll take action.

Responding to pain, rather than reacting, is an opposite that's correlated with lower stress and less pain. Observe reactivities to pain from many perspectives. Analyze reactivity objectively to uncover effective opposites. Test those opposites to find responsible solutions. The rewards are clearer thinking, better relationships, less pain and stress, less illness....

Step back and accept feeling pain. Turn down its stress and respond, rather than react. Clear your mind, rather than allowing long-term stress to cloud it up. Perform chronic pain control techniques. Consciously activate endorphins and pain control pathways to take control away from the brain's pain-creating pathways.

As discussed earlier, you cannot flee from pain, so fleeing is not the answer. Don't run from pain. Face it and embrace it, without anger. Stress gives pain power, so do not feed it stress. Do the opposite.

Pain is a lot like thoughts. It simply is. Go into pain and visualize it. Try to see the dimensions of pain; does it have shape, color, and texture? See it non-aggressively, all the way to its intangible core, to dissolve it and claim its power for your own. Its power is yours.

The nervous system adopts these new perspectives fairly quickly, so after a few attempts, the skill of accepting pain, as just another type of perception or type of thought, can become a powerful tool. Acceptance, rather than resistance, is an 'opposite' skill that takes power away from pain, giving that power to you. Through acceptance, allow the pain - do not fight it (fighting is stress). Acceptance has power over all manifestations of stress. Acceptance nullifies stress. Acceptance helps the mind become clear and alert, so it can move forward with appropriate responses. Acceptance helps open the way for pain-controlling endorphin pathways to work. At the same time, apply other MBPC techniques, such as laughter and the breath to evaporate pain.

This level of concentration for turning down the stress that accompanies pain takes energy and work while skills are still young. Strong intention always helps. Far less pain is the reward. Some pains take a few days to conquer (deep, intense spinal cord pain is an example) and that's okay. Along with the CBi Touch, all ten MBPC techniques can control even deep pain by manipulating the subjective conditions that sustain it.

Taking a deep breath to reduce pain is the opposite of not being able to catch your breath. Breathe deeply on purpose. When pain is so strong that it takes your breath away, successfully taking a deep breath requires conscious effort because it goes against the brain's instinctive reaction to increase pain. Laugh rather than cry. Smile rather than grimace.

The brain's default setting is to react with pain-supporting stress, emotions, and behaviors. Practice positive responses to pain, rather than reinforcing negative reactions. Change your perspectives to the opposite. Become mentally proactive, rather than reactive. Effective perspectives are always the opposite of the reactive, pain-supporting, default settings of the mind.

Relaxing during pain is an opposite because it goes against the brain's instincts. While trying to relax, the initial rise in stress may be obvious. To alter that, do not consult with the brain, as if to ask permission. Instead, reduce stress consciously with the full intention and the purpose of an objective response. Do not get frustrated. Do not force relaxation or stress will seep in. Rather than fighting tension or trying to argue with the mind to defend your desire to relax, or procrastinating to schedule a better time to do this, simply relax, absolutely relax, now. The pain wants to own you, but instead become the embodiment of confident, secure, lighthearted relaxation. This makes pain lose its grip.

The opposite of reaction to stress is to respond objectively and without judgment. Correct opposites don't support pain. Once the opposites that support less to no chronic pain become the new comfort zone of your altered reality, this type of pain control will make more sense. As you experience it, feel it, and witness it, you will fully believe it. Accepting the presence of pain cannot sustain the instinctive stress that supported it.

Release strong urges that cause you to stick with the old ways. Strengthen these new opposite thought, emotion, and behavioral perspectives, so they become second nature for you sooner than later. The more you practice MBPC techniques and the CBi Touch, the stronger and more effective those techniques will become. Don't force it; just allow and trust it.

The More You Use It, the Stronger It Gets.

Applying MBPC

For an example of how to apply these methods, I had the unfortunate opportunity to test MBPC techniques on a very serious source of pain. I fell on the sharp edge of a concrete step, and seriously bruised my sacroiliac joint and the surrounding 'tailbone' area. I was able to literally stop the pain, right away, using the CBi Touch, yet the actual healing took over a year and a half, while it remained swollen and inflamed for over two years.

I was occasionally made aware of how painful that condition should have been, had I not been controlling the pain from a bruised tailbone, by seemingly 'out of the blue' recurring nausea, uncontrollable and extreme reflexive grimacing in my face, suddenly not being able to catch my breath, and by sensations of being punched in the gut with reflexive doubling over.

Several times during the first three or four months, those symptoms happened repeatedly, randomly, and unexpectedly. Sharing my experience can teach others how to apply MBPC to effectively deal with some of the most intense pain-related symptoms, even if pain is being controlled.

'Out of the blue' doubling over often started by feeling as if a taut string were attached between my spine and a discrete, painful point at the back of my stomach. There was always the initial sharp burn at this imaginary 'point of attachment', followed by a powerful pull, as the imaginary string pulled my abdomen toward my spine. Then, the pulling sensation would change to pain radiating out in all directions. My spine would lurch backward, as my upper body bent forward, rolling me downward with tremendous force. It felt like someone kicked me in the stomach, causing me to double-over and fold in half.

It was alarming for my body to do this, seemingly without a reason. There was nothing to connect it to, except for the pain from the illusory, pulling string. I eventually realized I was actually doubling over in pain, even though the pain from my tailbone injury was silent; it wasn't even hurting. The absence of pain is why doubling over seemed to come from 'out of the blue'.

Sometimes doubling-over happened in very slow motion, without the string pull. It felt as if someone were steadily pushing me over from behind, pressing down against my shoulder blade area, slowly forcing me to bend forward, then I'd buckle at the knees and sink to the floor.

Also, my rib cage, facial muscles, and many other muscles throughout my body contracted or cramped, as my legs weakened and buckled in a span of about two seconds. It's possible to become so present and aware that you can notice and control nearly every aspect of it.

While being stressed and stuck in the doubled-over position, I tried to remember MBPC principles of opposites. My muscles were cramped, so I fully relaxed to enable standing up. I could not catch my breath, so I overcame that to breathe. The deep breath helped my facial muscles relax, so the tense grimacing could stop.

I smiled. Continuing slow, deep, conscious breaths on purpose, with smiles to turn on endorphin, plus relaxation, helped me end each doubling-over episode.

Nausea, doubling over with the kick in the gut, not being able to breathe, and intense facial grimacing may accompany an intensely painful injury. These behaviors can occur independent of pain because they and pain originate from different regions of the brain.

I am grateful that I was not suffering from tremendous pain in addition to the occasional nausea and doubling-over, while the tailbone slowly healed. I am sure the pain would have been tremendous.

Through my experience and observations, now you know how to apply opposites and MBPC techniques to handle cramping and doubling-over, if that ever happens to you. MBPC does not affect nausea, but fortunately there are effective nausea medications.

There is another important application of MBPC that could save a life. Hip injuries in the elderly can be life threatening. A severely injured or arthritic hip can cause a stronger effect on the brain than even doubling over. It can cause a type of depression that challenges the will to live. It feels as if each cell is telling all of the other cells to give up and let go. That is a terrifying realization and it zaps all of your energy. I understand how many succumb. I found that MBPC concepts help us convince ourselves that the severe depression and lack of will to live are being caused by biochemical reactions in the brain and that the brain has it wrong. The entire body is not actually as bad off as the hip makes it seem and this too shall pass. During that time of darkness, physics and biochemistry lead to mental misinterpretations and misperceptions in the cortex that make false claims. Remember that it's just an injured hip; the whole world has not changed. Stress is too elevated. Practice MBPC to reduce the stress. Breathe. Relax every muscle fiber. Continue on until the doctor can correct the condition. Repeat over and over, "This too shall pass. It's just a silly brain, after all." Life is so much brighter on the other side, which is closer than you think. Resist the darkness.

Invisible and intangible, yet intense perceptions of pain are susceptible to Mindfulness-based Pain Control techniques. In the case of abnormal chronic pain, which has no useful purpose, it is very fortunate that we can control it using our understanding of the brain and mind. Understanding the facts about how pain works, which represent what really matters about perceptions of pain, helps us prioritize those facts over the instincts of the mind in order to control pain responsibly, following a proper diagnosis, and with a doctor's permission.

Prioritize Matter Over Mind.

The Big Picture

Excluding grief and the full-blown stress of sudden imminent danger, we have more control over our emotions than we think. We can typically choose to feel relaxed or stressed simply by controlling or selecting the thoughts and beliefs we have at any given moment.

We usually look only at the surface of reality, only at the surface of what goes on around us. We think something 'outside' of us makes us feel the way we do. We are convinced we need a reason to smile, a reason to be happy, that we need something to take away the pain, or that we need something else to cause the feelings of fulfillment and satisfaction we 'think' we lack.

We must realize at a deeper level, that the same biochemicals and cells, and the same neural pathways in the brain that help us visualize and focus intensely, plus the endorphin pathways that give us lighthearted and enthusiastic feelings, which can control pain and our stress levels enough to stop them, none of these cells ever leave our body. They are always there. They are there for us to use any and every time we choose.

The biochemicals and their reactions inside our bodies do not 'know' if something outside of us has provided a sufficient 'reason' to feel the way we do. They are just chemicals, biochemicals; they are life's chemicals. They react according to the laws of physics.

Going up a few levels of complexity, through our increased understanding and awareness, we can exercise 'choice' in an instant to turn on endorphins and pleasure centers, if only because we now know this option is always available. We can do it in an instant, just as we can succumb to being stressed out in an instant.

Certainly, something on the outside can initiate feelings of satisfaction or dissatisfaction to be created inside of us. But we can choose to control the switch, and we do not need to wait for some external reason to flip the switch on for controlling our emotions and to control pain. We just flip it on. Change your mind-set and flip your state of mind from reactive to responsive, from stress all the way over to joy.

All of these techniques are powerful tools. They are waiting within your brain and body. Use them to create your experiences in life. Use them to control the aspects of mind that you can control. Enhance your well-being.

CB Intrinsic Touch and MBPC Combined

Applying MBPC and CBi Touch techniques provide all the tools adults need for responding with a clear mind and for allowing the normal acute pain-now/no-pain-later pathways, the opposite of abnormal chronic pain pathways, to be re-established through neuroplasticity.

Combining the Touch and MBPC together further enriches every experience and increases enthusiasm for us to improve overall well-being and succeed with chronic pain control.

We could say that using the CBi Touch with MBPC creates a positively Positive-Feedback Loop, because the synergy between decreasing stress and pain positively increases positive feelings, an optimal state of mind for improves health, controls chronic pain, re-establishes normal pain patterns, promotes gain-in-function for muscles and glands, and enriches one's quality of life.

The synergy between MBPC and the Touch is mind-blowing. It is the best way to simultaneously activate endorphin pathways from the Top-Down and Bottom-Up; together they activate endorphins throughout the entire body. They utilize neuroplasticity for long-term, beneficial change to normalize pain control processes.

All areas of the nervous system that prevent the perception of most forms of pain are being turned on all at once. As with scratching an itch for relief, the body and mind have solutions for lessening aberrant pain. Just as acute pain helps the body monitor conditions and minimize further injury, in an effort to protect our body's health, the nervous system also comes with intrinsic and natural methods for appropriately controlling pain.

Together, they are extremely successful at also reducing emotional pain and stress. Through endorphins, the nervous system reduces the severity of the long-term stress that accompanies excessive pain, significantly reducing the ill effects stress would have on the mind/body/spirit. These natural, intrinsic solutions are ever present, patiently waiting for us to use them.

Paradigm Shifts Are Powerful.

Become Empowered.

Methods for Controlling Chronic Pain

Smile
Relax
Socialize
Visualize
Feel Joyful
Be Accepting
Paradigm Shift
Feel Enthusiastic
Feel Lighthearted
Exercise to Ease Pain
Don't Focus on the Pain
Relax Every Muscle Fiber
Concentrate On Real Goals
Slow Deep Breaths Cancel Pain
Effective Perspectives Reduce Pain
Stimulated Light Touch Neurons Kill Pain
Smile/Laughter Reduce Stress -> Reduce Pain
Touch On Endorphins for Local Bottom-Up Control
Switch On Endorphins for Broader Top-Down Control
Use CB Intrinsic Techniques for Healthier
Mind/Body/Spirit
Alter Your Reality

Part IV

PARTNERSHIPS
IN
PAIN CONTROL

Tips for Significant ... Others

Over the decades and in different ways, those around me also struggled significantly with my pain. Writing Part IV has helped me reflect back, analyze some of the short comings, and sort out ways for improvement.

Others (**significant** other, family members, friends, healthcare professionals, and **others**) need to identify with the pain somehow. They need to know how to help in effective ways, see some progress for positive feedback, and build relationships that both gives and receives.

For others to understand the pain we are going through, we try to describe what that pain actually feels like. When I was very young, I described my first hernia as an erupting volcano with lava burning and tearing apart my chest. As I aged, my descriptions became general and vague; it really hurts, it's deep or sharp, or it aches. General descriptions help the other person judge the type of pain, but it isn't personalized.

For those around me, it was frustrating, day in and day out, to realize they couldn't help, they didn't know what to do differently, and the pain just kept coming back. It was exhausting. What were they supposed to do?

Sometimes relationships and respect are lost due to chronic pain. As months turn into years, at work or at home, giving up on being able to help, after trying for so long without success, with resentment and frustration building, in some cases, wishing the pain would go away turns into wishing that person would just go away.

Are there ways to offer support that actually help?

Having chronic pain most of my life, plus conditions that periodically cause relentless, recurring acute pain, I understand from the perspective of those suffering from pain. As someone who has also tried to help others experience less pain, I understand it from the support side, too. Perhaps I can help your efforts become more effective for helping your loved one, friend, coworker, or patient/client experience less pain, while building your relationships with skillful teamwork, shared feelings, empathy, compassion, and resilience against frustration.

Six Ways to Improve Support

1. Apply the CBi Touch
2. Apply MBPC Techniques
3. Stress Is Contagious
4. Acknowledging PC's Pain
5. Beliefs and Behaviors
6. It Takes a Village

It is important to learn all of the CB Intrinsic techniques, so common understanding will strengthen skills for both of you, increasing your effectiveness for pain reduction as a team. CBi techniques will help you personally, too, since pain visits all of us at some point. And skillful application of MBPC improves mind/body/spirit health overall for whomever practices it.

Apply the CB Intrinsic Touch

For brevity and differentiation's sake:
    SO = Significant ... Others (generic he)
    PC = Pain Controllers   (generic she)

Being able to apply the Intrinsic Touch is a very effective way to help reduce anyone's physical pain, including your own. It sooths away stress. It is a tactile sensation that feels really good; some say it feels sensual. Following the instructions in Part II and by practicing your skills regularly, you can master the CBi Touch.

To know how long to apply the Touch, ask PC to tell you when the pain has either stopped or is significantly reduced. Once that is achieved, stop your application of the Touch for that session.

Make sure you can apply the four Touch types: mosquito, spider, chipmunk, and snake. Begin with the mosquito or spider, practicing that method over time, until PC's nervous system has learned to respond to your touch, before advancing to the chipmunk and snake.

Reaching a significant reduction in pain could happen the instant SO and PC begin working together, but more often it can take 15 minutes for a new SO relationship. Over time, that interval decreases as SO's touch and PC's nervous system's response meld. To progress to the chipmunk and snake methods, apply the Touch only until the pain subsides. Learn everything you can in Part II about performing the Intrinsic Touch.

Apply MBPC Techniques

Part III teaches skills that not only enhance the effectiveness of the Touch for pain control, but also lower stress levels, calm instinctive pain processing, and train mental processes to turn on endorphins throughout the body to reduce pain long-term. Those skills are healthy and can be used in all situations.

As far as helping PC more effectively, practice Mindfulness-based Pain Control (MBPC) skills together. These skills are not intuitive and require a change in thought processes. Understanding the rationale behind MBPC techniques will improve your support and enhance your probability of success. Read and absorb the concepts in Part III. Talk with PC about it. You won't be able to personally determine if the techniques work until you use them with your own pain (which might not happen for a while). You must rely on PC's feedback to know how effective your skills are against pain.

Practice MBPC together. Plan distractions and work on goals together. Smile and laugh, feel lighthearted and enthusiastic about even the smallest things when you are together. The 'relax every muscle' exercise is healthy for everyone as a meditation, whether or not there is pain. It feels good all on its own.

Include being aware of your breaths. Some may want to visualize together what your lives will be like 6 weeks or 6 months from now, when pain control releases both of you to enjoy life more fully again.

Be accepting and patient with PC's pain and your abilities to help. Teamwork does more than optimize your support of PC's progress toward mastering pain control skills. Partnership in exercising CBi techniques nurtures a healthier relationship, and minimizes frustrations as your abilities to help improve, while successes increases.

Stress Is Contagious

Chronic pain has a lot of stress associated with it. Everyone involved experiences that stress; everyone.

PCs Experience Elevated Stress Levels

Sometimes the stress from suffering through a chronic pain episode is like having your legs covered with biting fire ants, and you can't get them off fast enough.

If you can't imagine a fire ant attack, the scene in "Outlander" (Starz and Netflix) when Caitriona Balfe's character, Claire Randall, is attacked by fire ants comes close (Season 3, Episode 11). Caitriona's skillful acting made the searing ant stings look believable.

Watching that scene reminded me of the time my best friend (2 years old) and I (3.5 years old) were stung, bitten, and attacked by hordes of fire ants coming out of the fire ant mound we were standing on. Too young to know about fire ant mounds or how to respond rationally, i.e., run, we panicked, froze, and stared at the front door of my house, standing side by side, bare-legged in little girl dresses, crying and screaming. My brothers ran outside to scoop us up. It was obviously quite traumatic since she and I remember it vividly to this day.

Covered in ants, screaming in pain, both standing on the top of a fire ant mound, not knowing how to make the pain stop is how intense chronic pain becomes sometimes. Stress and anxiety peak, as in mountain peak, with the pain, while panic takes over. Hopefully, someone's brothers will run outside to help.

Stress and anxiety levels rise to match pain levels. That stress automatically shuts down the regions of the brain responsible for logical thinking, assessing a situation clearly, making sound risk/benefit judgments, processing the passage of time, recognizing one's own denial, believing in reward regardless of risk, believing (irrational) actions are justified and sound, acting impulsively, and experiencing lapses in the 'ability to think'. High pain and high stress lead to low cognition. It is set up that way in the brain, unfortunately.

PC may believe she is thinking clearly and that her stress levels are low and contained, yet she can't tell that she is in denial of possibly off the charts stress. She could be stubborn and resistant to SO's advice. SO's suggestions may make her even more stressed. She could reach her limit and panic.

The way stress and pain interact is complex. An understanding, patient SO, skilled in MBPC techniques can do a world of good to help PC remember her skills for lowering her stress. PCs need SOs to help them walk off of the fire ant mound or climb down from the mountain peak.

SO becomes the coach, draws on his experiences, applies his CBi skills, remains calm, and uses gentle firmness when necessary to protect PC from the danger her high stress and low cognition levels represent.

SO gently reminds PC of the techniques he thinks could help the specific situation they are in. They practice those skills together, SO helping PC through the tough spots. Striving for a calm and caring attitude, rather than using an agitated or forceful coaching style, SO helps PC's stress levels diminish to some degree.

Calm is contagious. Keep your calm to help PC catch it from you. Resist catching PC's stress as much as possible, while helping her recognize the best decisions and actions to take. SO's input is critical in these times to protect PC from acting on bad decisions.

I recently had another experience that demonstrates how truly important SOs are. It's a great example of how an SO's calm, clear mind can save a PC (me) from making a potentially grave mistake.

An excessively painful (12 out of 10), post-surgical infection began one late afternoon. The pain was so intense that I carefully removed the surgical bandages to see what was going on. There was a long, red, angry-looking rash a few inches away from and running parallel to my 3-day old incision. I spread an antibiotic salve over the rash immediately, hoping that would heal the infection.

I knew to abide by the CBi rule to NEVER apply the Touch to an untreated, undiagnosed infection, no matter how painful it was. Since the bandages were meant to stay on, and I did put them back on, pain was the only way I could monitor the infection's progress.

The next morning, after a very painful night, I checked the rash again. After noticing it had spread and was inching closer to the incision, I applied more salve. Late that afternoon, I told my friend Janet, who stopped by for a visit, about the infection, saying I was planning to give the salve another 24 hours to work, rather than bugging the doctor about it.

The fact that the infection was spreading very quickly and that the pain was through the roof helped Janet (now an SO) realize I wasn't thinking rationally. She mentioned I was looking ill and tried to intervene. Janet suggested I call the doctor's office now, instead of waiting until tomorrow. She told me that waiting until the next day might not be healthy, and that I could live to regret waiting.

She related a personal story about when she waited too long to complain to her doctor's office about a problem she had. Waiting caused serious complications that she continues to regret to this day. I remained in denial about needing to call my doctor, but Janet didn't give up.

Realizing it was essential for me to reduce my stress level so I could think more rationally, Janet remained calm and did not become frustrated or overly stressed. She talked about facts without interjecting negative emotions.

Janet pointed out that it's easy to call the doctor's office, and that I wouldn't be bugging him, since doctoring is what he does for a living. She pointed out that since the infection spread during the night, I should consider how much it would spread by tomorrow. She implored me to consider whether I could afford to take that risk. Was the salve even helping?

Eventually, Janet calmly and rationally convinced me to call my doctor. The doctor's office scheduled an appointment for 'as soon as I could get there'.

The pain was beyond my tolerance. When the doctor's nurse (SO) took off my bandages, the infection had spread even further and there were blisters. My doctor (SO) prescribed antibiotics and told me he wanted me to start taking them immediately. He warned me that if I couldn't start them that evening or waited until tomorrow to start them, I could end up in the hospital needing IV antibiotics.

It was nearly evening, and I was a town away from my drugstore, which was going to close soon. Thank goodness for cell phones. I called ahead to be sure my friends behind the drugstore counter (SOs) received the prescription and told them my Uber driver was rushing me there now. We arrived with only fifteen minutes to spare before they would have closed. My Uber driver (SO) went in to get the prescription for me, out of the goodness of his heart.

I knew to never apply the Touch or MBPC to my infection pain. It was at a 12 out of 10 for about 60 hours total, taking 4 more days to gradually stop. The infection itself continued spreading until it reached and went beyond the incision, but starting the antibiotic pills in the nick of time kept the infection from becoming septic.

I avoided being hospitalized for IV antibiotics, which depended on all of my SOs helping me that day; my friend Janet, my doctor and nurse, my kind and concerned Uber driver, and my friends at the drugstore who worked extra fast to fill that prescription in time. Thank you, SOs! PCs around the world thank their SOs!

SOs play a critical role in improving PCs' outcomes every day, all across the globe. It's the little things. Being skilled in MBPC provides critical skills for SOs. Knowing how to apply the Touch, and especially when NOT to apply it, is critical. Being able to help PC control and improve her situation is an honorable and wonderful way to help someone you care for.

As Janet put it, "It was a good day for both of us."

And yes, it is possible; there are ways that SOs can offer support that actually, really helps.

SOs Experience Elevated Stress Levels

PCs are not the only ones who feel stressed because chronic pain is controlling their lives. Depending on the relationship, some SOs also struggle with PC's pain that runs constantly in the background of their lives, too.

Perhaps for married couples, the quality of life for both are negatively impacted. Perhaps the number of times they are able to do something together as a couple is reduced. Doing less things together may or may not seem like a problem, but it will take a toll over time. Chronic pain can be hard on a marriage. The same may be true for work relationships, all relationships, perhaps.

Be social - don't isolate. Make lists of what you used to love or enjoy doing together, categorized by what you can do now and what hope to do eventually. Practicing the Touch can make it easier to do more activities. Start doing things again together, but take it slowly. PC may need to build her energy stores. Go at her pace.

MBPC can help both of you reduce PC's pain and reduce stress for both of you to better maintain a healthy relationship. As pain plays less and less of a role, and the fear of being more active fades away more and more, look back in a few months to notice how many more things you are doing together as a couple. Notice how much more you are interacting with your friends. Look at all the good memories you now are making together. Notice how much fuller life is becoming.

Soak it up. Feel the stress releasing you to live your lives again. Accept and enjoy the fruits of practicing pain control together.

SOs Sometimes Reach a Limit

Yet there are days that SO does not feel supportive. SOs get tired of endless pain, too. Situations surrounding pain can get to any SO sometimes. Stress and tension rise. Frustrations rise. Tempers may flare. SOs may just want to give up. May I make a suggestion?

Pick up this book and go for a drive to your local sanctuary or lock yourself in the basement and read. Breathe. You are not able to see it sometimes, but your help is crucial, and all that you do is appreciated. Still, sometimes SOs get stressed out. MBPC can help.

Getting stressed is instinctive. It's okay. Feel it for a few minutes and then tell your mind that's enough. Start reading Part III again. Let the pages take you away and remind you of all the ways we can control our stress. Remember what stress will do if you don't control it. And stress in contagious. Learn how to release your stress so it won't make PC's pain and stress rise along with yours.

The only type of stress that is healthy is 'short-term' stress. That type of stress helps you dash out of the way of a massive, falling tree when you have only a millisecond to get out of its way, or lift a car off of a person trapped under it from an accident. The clear mind, focused attention, and superhuman speed, agility, and strength come with that sudden burst of stress (adrenalin or epinephrine), which is good. But long-term stress is very destructive for your body, mind, and spirit, due to elevated cortisol levels long-term. Endorphin stops that.

MBPC helps you reduce long-term stress for whatever the cause. Since stress is contagious, try not to give it to each other. If you are both able, practice MBPC stress reduction skills together. Let her help you reduce your stress, as you have been selflessly helping her reduce her pain. It's her turn to help you, now. Share the gift.

Remember stress is contagious, long-term stress is harmful, and MBPC helps PC/SO reduce stress together.

Acknowledging PC's Pain

PC and SO relationships around pain have a range of complexities. With over a billion PCs around the world and many more SOs, we can't imagine all the issues that might arise, but we can share a few. I hope addressing some common issues will help improve communications and relationships for PCs and SOs.

Doubting PC's Pain

It's basic human nature to look for proof supporting reasons for pain, otherwise doubts become an issue.

Doubting PC's pain is not an issue when SO knows PC well, perhaps witnessed the sudden onset of pain, has unconditional empathy for someone who looks like they are in pain, and/or knows that the pain tracks well with PC's diagnosed condition.

When SO doesn't know PC well, doubting PC's pain is not an issue if there's a diagnosis or if SO can see the reason for the pain (swelling, compound fracture, open wound), and/or SO has understanding or experience with the same pain and condition, as is found amongst members of pain support groups.

Doubt is not an issue for doctors and nurses relying on their professional experience for assessing patients' pain. For example, PCs use a 1-10 ranking and descriptor words (sharp, dull, deep, ache, burning) to help doctors and nurses assess both the pain level and types of pain. Their trained eye recognizes pain symptoms that are consistent with a condition(s). We could say that there are Six Factors of Proof that help SOs not doubt PCs.

Six Factors for Proof
- Knowing and Trusting PC
- Unconditional Empathy
- Visible Signs - Injured Tissues
- Having a Diagnosed Condition
- Personal Experience - Shared Condition/Pain
- Education About the Diagnosed Condition

Naturally, when none of those factors are met, SO may have doubt. In worst case scenarios, given billions of PC/SO relationships in the world, occasionally an SO's doubts morphs into a false opinion that is taken as truth. Doubting morphs into believing that PC's pain is not real.

Chronic pain sufferers without a diagnosis often experience this. It is frustrating for SO's and infuriating for PC's. Doubt reduces the quality of the SO/PC relationship. Frustration, conflict, and resentment over chronic pain validation can sully even the best PC/SO relationships.

Relationships under those conditions can become harmful on many levels. The added stress alone increases the unpleasantness, intensity, frequency, and duration of PC's pain. Doubt at the least hinders or prevents an SO's ability to offer productive support. And yet, we know SOs do want to help. That creates more stress, which makes it even harder.

One of the most sorrowful aspects of suffering from chronic pain for PCs is not being believed. PCs must find solace in believing that no one intentionally doubts them. It's part of the wide spectrum of human nature. Feeling upset about this doubt raises anxiety and stress, further complicating and worsening PCs' situation.

Analyzing the situation from both SOs' and PCs' perspectives may help those relationships. Starting with the first factor for proof, mend the relationship. PC/SO must get to know and trust each other more. Commit more quality time with questions and active listening. Take extra time to Listen. Work together to nurture openness, honesty, and integrity. Remember that it is difficult for PC to convince SO of her pain, and likewise, it is difficult for SO to internalize and feel her pain.

Pain Lacks Recall

Years ago, a pediatrician spoke with me jokingly about our inability to remember pain, saying that if we had perfect recall for intense pain, no women would go through childbirth more than once. In addition to impacting the global population, the fact that pain does not have memory contributes to doubting PC's pain.

There is not a place in the brain that stores memory of pain. We remember our thoughts and emotions about pain because we can store thoughts and emotions in the brain. We can share thoughts and prove thoughts with words. Writing down words helps us remember thoughts we might have forgotten. We can cause thoughts to return by re-reading our words. The exact thoughts.

But we cannot store pain in the brain. We cannot share it or make it return at will because pain is a present moment thing. When it does exist, it only exists now.

Due to the lack of recall, believing how intense pain is can be difficult for SOs and even PCs. Intense pain is literally unbelievable, even as you experience it.

Because it reaches such inhumane levels, we'd think no one could ever forget it. We believe we remember pain, but we're only left with our thoughts and emotions surrounding it. Details about pain itself are as sketchy and hard to hold on to as those of a bad dream, the moment we wake up. So even PCs are shocked by its unfathomable depth and strength, and find it difficult to believe, each time it returns.

Perhaps not being able to recall our own pain is what makes it difficult to imagine in others. And without SO having experienced intense pain, it is impossible for him to know or imagine it, whether for one's self or others.

To offer quality support, it helps SOs to be able to identify with what it's like to endure prolonged, chronic pain. Empathy benefits from understanding and prior experience. Lacking experience or empathy puts SOs at a disadvantage. It might help those SOs to walk in PCs' shoes for a moment.

Mental Trickery

The pain is real for PCs, but it's not real for SOs. Getting on the same page is crucial for saving the PC/SO relationship. Lacking sufficient factors for proof, communication is the best hope for dispelling doubt.

As mentioned earlier in the book, pain and thoughts are similarly perceived in the cortex of the brain. Similar to the way a fragrance or song can bring back old memories and transport us to a different place and time, revisiting thoughts and emotions linked to past pain helps us travel back in time to reflect on past pain experiences. Revisiting their own pain experiences could help SOs empathize with PCs' pain. Thoughts, emotions and imagining past SO pain can provide a new way to help relieve SOs' doubts.

We've all seen a good movie (or read a good book) that could virtually transport us into its characters' lives. We would momentarily forget our own lives in exchange for the thoughts, emotions, and actions of the characters on the screen. The world of light projected onto the screen actually seems to exist in real-time.

Minds are easily tricked. The key is for our thoughts to match our emotions (i.e., no doubting), while our imagination remains focused on the seemingly real world projected on that scene, now, in the present moment. That's how minds work. Seeing is believing.

Virtual reality (VR) therapy convinces the mind so thoroughly that seeing a painful arm move and work painlessly through the VR headset makes the mind believe the real arm has no pain. Minds are easy to trick.

It seems there should be a way to trick the mind into appreciating someone else's pain, so how do we do it?

If I were to say a pain is killing me, you get the idea that it is intense, but without already knowing intense pain, an SO couldn't imagine what that feels like, and certainly not well enough to identify with it or appreciate it. If I were to say this is a really deep, dull pain, you understand that only if you have experienced a deep, dull pain before.

Even if you could imagine deep and dull, that only describes the type of pain. Knowing the type of pain does not transport the SO into his past experience of it. Understanding the pain type isn't enough to give a sense of it. Simulated pain might awaken empathy and relieve doubt.

It could help for the mind to visualize that it is in a painful situation right now. SO could experience a mental movie, guided by PC's detailed storyline. If the storyline can help SO attach a similar, personal, past pain experience to PC's pain, the thoughts and the emotions welling up inside SO may trigger what it was like for SO to suffer that similar pain in his past. That renewed understanding and experience could lead to trust, understanding, and empathy. This may be all that is lacking. This may relieve doubt.

PC takes the lead in this exercise. Her role is to find a storyline that will indirectly lead SO closer to understanding and not doubting her pain. PCs need to come up with a storyline for the mental movie, but it will not be about PC's story. PC chooses a storyline that is designed to help SO remember his own story, make his own mental movie in his mind about his past pain experiences, to identify with his own pain again.

To be clear, SO can never feel PC's pain (even if they share an identical injury at the same time - pain is perception, interpreted and created by each brain). So, having SO feel PC's pain is not the goal. Also, SO does not need to share PC thoughts and emotions related to her pain. SO simply needs to access his own thoughts and emotions surrounding his own past pain that is similar to PC's current pain.

PC must compare her current chronic pain(s) with similar acute pains SO may have felt in the past. She considers what incident most people have experienced that would have caused pains similar to hers. Perhaps accidentally hitting a finger, instead of the nail, with a hammer feels something like her chronic pain. She checks to see that SO experienced it in the past. He did.

Remembering SO's experience of hitting his finger with a hammer may be the right storyline and PC will guide the progression of scenes to help SO recall his experience.

PC must allow SO's mind the space and time it needs to travel back in time, select and set the scene for his mental movie, as he is guided by her storyline.

While SO becomes immersed in the storyline, listening to PC's voice and following along, PC's storyline gently guides SO's brain and mind. This is literally a type of meditation. Both focus solely on this.

SO's mind will re-experience his story, filling it in with memories of his past hammering experiences. It takes time to search in the recesses of his mind to recall details of his past situations. PC must observe SO, allowing him to travel at his own speed. SO's hammer experience may be vague at first, but as PC helps him recall the details, SO can remember it more clearly.

PC could expand her storyline to simulate the long-term component of her chronic pain, helping it apply to her current pain a bit more.

PC selected the hammer storyline only because it is a fairly common experience that links to pains which feel similar to her current pain. PC's thoughts and emotions about her pain, or even her pain itself, cannot transfer to SO. The storyline itself and SO's ability to become one with that are all that are needed to transport SO back to his past experience, thoughts, and emotions related to his hammering and smashed finger pain. For PC to direct or shape his mental movie with her thoughts and emotions would not be effective for SO at this time.

To better understand what I mean, let's say SO is coming up on his 30th high school graduation anniversary. He would like to get on a plane and go the party, but he has to stay home for work. PC wants to help him celebrate it at home with fun decorations, some of his high school memorabilia, and a musical trip back in time. PC listened to country music when she went to in high school, so she downloaded plenty of country western songs.

SO listened to jazz in high school. To be taken back to the good ole, high school days, SO would need to listen to jazz. He needs to replay his memories, not PC's; try as hard as she may, PC's memories can't take him there.

Pain is kind of like that. We cannot feel another person's pain. The thoughts and emotions that link to painful experiences of the past are contained within each person's mind. Substituting another's pain-related thoughts and emotions won't work.

We need to feel our own emotions while watching, listening to, or reading a well told story. The way we 'live' a story will be based on our own past experiences. It is important for our own emotions to match our thoughts.

PC's storyline helps SO remember his own thoughts and emotions that are connected to his past experiences with a pain that is similar to PC's. Connecting SO's experiences and emotions to PC's can help reduce SO's doubt, improve trust, understanding and empathy. Hopefully, SO will feel that his support is more effective and rewarding, and notice that his attempts at helping feel less frustrating.

Making Mental Movies

We are interested in doing this exercise because SO has doubts, since he lacks experience with intense or relentless pain like PC's, and is having a hard time relating to it. Perhaps not enough of the Six Factors have been met, or PC and SO think a mental movie could be fun. And SO truly wants to be as helpful as possible. Whatever the reasons, relationships benefit from a mental movie.

The first step for putting the storyline together is for PC to analyze her pain(s). She must imagine what I call its dimensions, textures, colors, intensities, rhythms, and its mixtures of every characteristic and nuance. She must fearlessly embrace her pain's full reality.

Using effective perspectives, go deeply into the pain to see it all the way to its intangible core (p. 160). Face it, hold it, analyze it. Sometimes PC's pain may diminish while doing this exercise, but focus on every nuance while pain remains. Write it all down and make a list.

If PC's pain is in her neck, and she uses neck pain for her storyline, but SO hasn't had a pain in his neck, that storyline won't be very effective. PC must figure out which common experiences she and SO share that cause pains similar to her chronic pain. Many conditions create similar or the same type(s) of pain. PC must build the story around another reason for a similar pain to the one she experiences from her neck.

For example, a common experience that creates a pinched nerve type of pain in the neck could be a sudden jab in the heal by a small, sharp piece of gravel in a shoe as we walk. That's sharp and painful enough to make us stop immediately to remove it before continuing on.

If stepping on sharp pieces of gravel in the shoe feels similar to her current neck pain, that could be PC's main storyline. Let's say it is and help SO make a mental movie. This works best as a guided meditation and not a conversation or debate. PC speaks, while SO closes his eyes better visualization and concentrated imagination. SO nods each time he is ready for PC to move to the next step.

PC creates the storyline and sets the stage:

PC makes sure SO has experienced walking with a sharp piece of gravel in his shoe. (If not, it's easy enough to go outside and try it.) Ask SO to silently remember some of the details about those pain sensations and try to remember what he did about it. As SO builds his movie set, give him time to reflect back to remember what the environment was like, where he was walking, what shoes he had on, etc. He could describe it to PC as he settles in.

PC extends remembering into imagination:

Ask SO to imagine what it might be like if he couldn't remove the sharp gravel and had to continue walking. SO imagines that his heal is continually being jabbed with sharp, acute pain. SO gets into his movie character to 'live' the part.

PC expands the story further:

Now SO must imagine the shoe has at least 20 sharp pieces of gravel in it, yet he must continue walking. He can't stop to shake out the stones.

SO must imagine both shoes have sharp gravel in them, and he must run. The pain won't stop and is intense. Now the pain is very intense.

Could SO imagine collapsing because the pain is so intense? The pain is insanely intense, and his feet are quite injured. But he has to continue running.

From the analysis of her own pain earlier:

Choosing descriptive terms or words that PC's pain analysis revealed earlier, ask if SO's imagined, acute foot pain might also feel _fill in the blank_ .

PC substitutes chronic in place of acute:

Ask SO to imagine how his life might change if he had gravel in his shoes every day and night, every time he walked. (PC is careful to allow enough time for SO to reflect, since his mental movie scenes are created at his pace. Give SO's imagination time to evolve. SO nods.)

PC could expand the experience further:

Image what would it be like walking up and down the aisles at the grocery store for an hour and a half with gravel in both shoes. Imagine that your feet remained relentlessly painful, even with his shoes off, while resting with his bare feet elevated. Still the pain. Imagine the sharp pain continuing as he tries to sleep, and that being sound asleep was the only relief he could find. Feel that pain in your feet, SO.

Post mental movie and the session is finished:

Share with SO that PC experiences similar pains in her neck, under her shoulder blades, across her shoulders, and down her arms, night and day, every day, and that she can't stop to remove the gravel from her shoes.

That is just one example for how PC and SO could use a meditative story (vs a conversational story) to create virtual, common experiences for shared understanding. It provides a type of self-evidence because the detailed, self-reflective, meditative storyline allows SO's mind to reach back in his past to find truth from his own pain-related thoughts and emotions. Reading this section in and of itself may help PC and SO get on the same page.

Subconsciously, PC's pain may have been in doubt for SO, but not as much any longer. To some degree, SO can imagine the pain he'd feel if he were in PC's shoes. He can better identify and empathize with PC's situation. This understanding, through virtual experience, offers insights that are difficult to gain any other way.

Beliefs and Behaviors

How do I improve my effectiveness as an SO?

With the billions of PC/SO relationships, I suppose most SOs ask that question at some point. We are literally blind to how our beliefs and behaviors negatively impact our PC/SO relationship, so issues arise.

Doctors and nurses spend years in school and decades practicing medicine, perfecting their skills to offer their best efforts for helping patients. Families, friends, and significant others also hope to do their best for their PCs. Why does it become so hard sometimes?

Being a great SO comes naturally for most. We rarely think to ask why. When I break it down to consider what makes being an SO effective, things like empathy and compassion come to mind. Diving a little deeper, many other elements contribute to SO effectiveness, too.

This list isn't complete, but effectiveness depends on topics we have already discussed, such as embracing intrinsic controls for chronic pain, having knowledge and understanding about PC's condition(s), remembering our own personal experiences with pain, being committed to healthy PC/SO relationships, and having a genuine appreciation for PC's situation. We could include the importance of learning how to ask questions rather than assuming to already know, examining hidden, subconscious expectations that we have, and resolving stubborn, uncomfortable conflicts to enhance and enrich the PC/SO relationship over time.

Nagging Assumptions

Family, friends, and significant others naturally make assumptions about PC's pain. Those assumptions combine to build a picture of what we think PC's pain is like, how it should progress, and how PC should behave.

SO may think, "It shouldn't still be like this. PC should have gotten over that by now. It isn't as bad as PC makes it out to be. If it were me, I'd still get stuff done and I wouldn't complain so much."

Those opinions are natural for SOs. It's human nature to base someone else's experiences on our own.

Without thinking about it or realizing it, assumptions are stated, and therefore, taken as unexamined fact. The problem with that is, without evidence, assumptions are opinions.

We have a right to our opinions, but to be responsible and accountable we must realize the consequences of acting on our opinions. And we must not be blind to our assumptions. We must be aware that we have these assumptions/opinions. We must question them.

Scientists are trained to question assumptions. They realize the true value of any assumption is that it points to the right questions to ask. Assumptions are questions without the question mark.

Stating an unquestioned assumption as a fact is so instinctive that turning an assumption from a statement into a question takes skill. Learning how to transform opinions and assumptions is essential. For pain control, the goal for an SO is to transform assumptions into questions, before instinctively uttering an accusation.

We know which assumptions these are. They tend to nag at us, increase stress levels, and sometimes make us angry. They make us feel frustrated, impatient, and a bit resentful toward PC. We want things to be better now, but they're not. Not only that, SO's help hasn't shown much progress lately, and trying to help feels futile.

PC/SO relationships based on assumptions lays a foundation of sand. Assumptions are not the answers. Instead, assumptions are used to show us which questions to ask. They are pointing to the right questions because the most uncomfortable assumptions that nag at us are begging us to step back, reflect, become aware, and resolve the issues that are formulating in the mind.

When we feel conflict about PC's pain and condition, we need to look deep inside to uncover whatever is begging for our attention. Turn opinions into questions.

To use assumptions effectively:
1. Remove the assumption's emotions.
2. Turn each assumption into questions.
3. Ask the questions.
4. Listen to PC's facts about her situation.
5. Ask more questions.
6. Get more evidence with (online) research.
7. Clarify your understanding with PC.
8. Understand it from PC's perspective.
9. Apply.
10. Support.
11. Nurture the PC/SO relationship.
12. Seek and grow with gratitude.

Addressing the Questions

Self-reflection is good. Rather than assuming the relationship is a bit edgy because of PC, SO must recognize that one of his subconsciously held, unnoticed assumptions or opinions is unintentionally causing conflict. SO's must be open to the possibility that he is blind to the ways their relationship is suffering from his mindset. Accept the possibility with an open mind.

Which opinions or assumptions about PC bug SO the most? Recognize them by the negative emotions; they feel bad. No matter how certain SO is about an opinion, turn it into a question anyway.

It's a difficult skill to learn since believing we know is a very strong instinct. Turn the opinion or assumption around and ask it as a question. Be open to the answer(s). Breathe and be prepared to accept. The facts you'd like to know, the answers your assumption/opinion begs for are the realities about PC's world, PC's facts.

Facts do not have emotions. They simply are. Our opinions and judgments add the emotions. We may react and feel emotions about facts, but facts themselves do not carry emotions within them. There is no need to add stress or emotions to defend facts. To understand the facts often requires explanation. Explanations don't need emotions, unless for emphasis or to gain attention.

SO turns his assumption's statement into a question, opens his mind to allow potentially feeling conflicted about the answer, steadies his mind to not react before understanding, and prepares to absorb a fact from a new perspective, PC's perspective.

PC must carefully consider her answers to SO's questions. Once she feels certain her answers are factual for her situation, PC clearly states her facts and tries not to blemish them with emotion. Emotions are not meant to become the focus. The facts and explanations speak for themselves. Just contemplate, state the facts, and calmly explain wherever there is misunderstanding.

For an example, let's use the first assumption listed in the second paragraph at the beginning of this section.

"It shouldn't still be like this."

PC's condition may be 'chronic' pain and chronic means the condition continues long-term. Or perhaps PC's condition is what is chronic, while its pain is acute and continually recurring. Regardless, we follow the same steps. With an open mind, we turn the assumption around to determine its underlying question:

"Should PC still be feeling this pain?"

That's a great question. Perhaps pains for PC's condition should have ended by now. Ask PC if she is also concerned by how long the pain is lasting. Maybe you can help PC in very significant ways. Research it.

Ask PC if there is something more you could do. Does she need to visit her doctor or need help with the CBi techniques? Would it help to practice with the techniques together? Investigate why PC is still feeling this pain and uncover ways you can work on it together.

To access some actual scientific research, visit a university library or search 'scholarly review articles' online. Using "*key phrase* review - scholarly articles" in a Google Chrome search, filtering the dates for relatively recent articles, learn all the facts you can about PC's condition. If you need keywords, talk about it with PC. She may have some ideas, and she could benefit from looking through the literature, too. Make it a team project.

Scientific 'review' articles present the latest findings with less detailed scientific jargon so more people can understand. If the scholarly articles contain buzz words or concepts that you don't understand, search online to understand those, too. It's all good. Keep digging until you understand as much as you need. Apply what you've learned to be able to help PC more effectively.

PC can also ask SO how she might help him feel less frustrated. PC can reverse this exercise by self-reflecting to make sure SO feels appreciated. SO's facts do not need emotions or defense. SO and PC only need understanding. PC must turn her assumptions and opinions into questions, and ask SO the questions with an open mind. This is conflict resolution through relationship building. SO/PC benefit from opening up.

Sometimes searching for answers to the questions, while discussing feelings and frustrations for better understanding, with minimal emotion, is sufficient for relationship building. Anything that relieves stressful, nagging doubts is healthy and worthwhile.

Negative assumptions feel uncomfortable, but they have value because they point you in the right direction and help both SOs and PCs ask the right questions. Don't guess with opinions. Ask for and understand the facts. Build a stronger, deeper PC/SO relationship.

Expectations

As you know, chronic pain control techniques allow someone to stop their pain for a period of time (minutes, hours, days, weeks, months, years).

We are so accustomed to equating an injury or medical condition with pain. When we go to the doctor's office complaining of a sprain or torn ligament, pain should be present. If you go to a doctor's appointment to complain about something that no longer hurts, it's possible you'd be sent home before seeing the doctor.

Pain and the condition seem to be one. When we have a sore throat, we know we are well or getting better if the throat stops hurting. If we have a bruise, we know the bruise is better once it stops hurting. If I have surgery, I know I'm healed once it stops hurting. No hurting equals healed. Not so with chronic conditions.

Having read this book, it is clear that pain and the injury or condition are not one, but they are intimately linked. What happens if we take pain away from a chronic condition, such as arthritis? Did we cure the condition?

If the sprained or torn ligament would normally hurt for a month or two, but we control the pain in the first week, did the injury heal that week? Does the injury heal every time you sleep and then recur again the minute you wake up? For short-term conditions, like strep throat, pain goes away as the illness heals. For long-term conditions, taking the pain away early is not a spontaneous cure. But, strangely, we may act like it is.

I bring this up because once PC doesn't hurt anymore, or for a significant period of time, SO must not forget that a chronic condition still exists. It is still as severe as the pain was indicating. When the pain is being skillfully controlled, a chronic condition still rages on.

If PC's hip is injured and the pain is controlled, even gone, PC still needs to take the stairs very carefully and perhaps still walk with a cane for balance and stability outdoors on uneven terrain. With the pain controlled, continue practicing all of the precautions inherent with the injury or condition. PC isn't in the clear. PC is just more comfortable and less stressed.

SOs are human and have expectations of others, just like anybody else. If PC is hurt, SO expects to see evidence of pain to tell how hurt PC is. If PC isn't in pain anymore, SO may expect PC to act as if all is well now.

Remember how a very serious injury may cause nausea and doubling over, even when the pain is controlled? PC may be controlling the pain, but other parts of the brain may be busy reacting to the injury or condition as if the pain were still there in full force.

SO needs to watch for signs that the condition is worsening, just as PC needs to be observant in the absence of her pain. If PC feels nauseous, or gets a fever, loses her appetite, becomes depressed for no obvious reason, and/or feels anxiety, restlessness, and/or a sense of urgency increases, remember that if she were not controlling her pain while having these symptoms, it would be assumed that the condition could be worsening. It would be obvious that she needs to see a doctor.

If worsening symptoms occur, remind PC that she must not apply MBPC or the Touch. PC must allow pain to continue if it returns, no matter how intense it is, so her doctor can use that to make a new diagnosis. It must be allowed to continue for the doctor's appointment. If the pain does not come back, that's okay. She still needs to see the doctor, based on other worsening symptoms.

If PC is not in pain during the doctor's appointment, help PC explain that you and she know how to control pain. Mention that the goal is to control her pain so PC can live a more comfortable life, regain whatever function is possible to regain, and reduce the negative effects of long-term stress. Mention the other symptoms from her worsening condition which indicate her pain would be intense, were she not controlling it. SO might show this book to the doctor and explain it a bit, to help medical professionals understand PC's lack of pain.

We believe we know how a person should act or behave, given their circumstances. It's human nature for us to subconsciously forget that when PC's pain is controlled, she still has a condition that needs care. Except for forms of neuropathy, remember that pain and its chronic condition are not one. For example, arthritis continues to deform and destroy with or without its pain. It would be nice for PC to be fully normal once her pain is gone, but that won't be the case for most conditions. The condition still needs to be monitored and corrected as soon as possible, whether there is pain or no pain. Expect that the condition remains. Remind yourself.

It Takes a Village

We have covered many topics related to our relationships with pain and stress throughout this book. Whether the condition has been, is about to be, or can't be diagnosed, there is always a real reason for chronic pain.

Medicine depends on technology and research, which have both come a long way and are works in progress, always. Not having a diagnosis could mean the right test hasn't been invented yet. Every condition for chronic pain that is currently undiagnosed will be discovered, characterized, and testable eventually.

Everyone's body/mind/spirit differs in various ways. Some differences are visible, while others are at the molecular level and invisible to our eyes. Nervous systems and experiences with pain vary among individuals. Each individual's experience with pain is 100% valid for that individual. Someone's pain does not have to be validated by or for anyone else for it to exist.

It is not up to others to judge, but rather to try to understand and help in effective ways that avoid creating further harm. Helping shouldn't include trying to make PC behave and believe according to SO's expectations and opinions about pain. SOs must release preconceptions to open their minds and be flexible enough to accept PC's version of pain. Using the techniques together, build mindful relationships based on integrity, honesty, trust, understanding, compassion, empathy, and cooperation.

Rather than moving passively from one day into the next, following wherever typically unobserved mindsets lead, awaken and use these healthy, stress reducing, pain controlling concepts to nurture and strengthen your PC/SO relationship.

1. Turn on endorphins to stop unnecessary pain, while accessing joy and bliss.
2. Resist directing life because healthy relationships do not emphasize power and control.
3. Rather than state opinions about how PC's pain should be, ask questions to dispel presumptions.
4. To lower stress levels and make decisions with a clearer mind, rather than fighting how things are, accept what is to respond, rather than react.
5. Due to innocent misunderstandings, countless imperfections in human nature, and the second law of thermodynamics, relationships become messy.
   a. Schedule routine PC/SO relationship maintenance.
   b. Resolve conflicts openly and constructively.
   c. Rejuvenate, realign, rebuild, and rejoice.
6. Use intrinsic pain control techniques appropriately.
7. Prioritize the condition's needs over pain control.
8. Regardless of how things are, live life with gratitude because we have options and true power over pain.

You Are Not Alone
It Takes A Village And
We Are All In This Together

Part V

PRECAUTIONS AND LIMITATIONS

Rules for the Road

The not-so-obvious downside to suffering from chronic pain includes the negative physical and emotional effects of the long-term stress it creates. Using CBi pain control techniques to help reduce chronic pain and its long-term stress is healthy for the physical well-being of mind, body, and spirit.

By stimulating endorphins to reduce pain and stress, the techniques improve sleep, organ health, and circulation, give a boost to the immune system, and re-energize enthusiasm for life.

This is also beneficial for every aspect of a person's life, including improved moods, personal relationships, emotional stability, clarity of thought and better decision making, and rejuvenated energy for work and play, which improve chances for living life as intended.

Yet inappropriate use poses a downside to pain control. Using the techniques inappropriately may cause serious harm, for example, prematurely stopping acute pain can be life threatening due to neglecting an injury.

The purpose for including this part of the teaching is cautionary. Using these techniques to inappropriately stop pain is tempting and deciding when to appropriately control pain is complicated. The brain's decision-making and impulse control centers are not fully developed until adulthood, but still there are risks for causing harm.

Whenever we are careless with pain control, unfortunate things can happen; worsening conditions, further injury, and/or unforeseen complications. For example, stopping the pain of a wasp, hornet, or bee sting, and receiving more stings painlessly could lead to sensitization due to the large amount of stinger-injected venom, and potentially serious allergic reactions to those types of stings later on. Pain is not the problem; the venom is. Feeling, observing, and interpreting pain is important for survival. Reemphasizing these warnings may help.

After years of practicing these techniques, my mind, perhaps instinctively, occasionally equates pain control with cure. Once pain is silenced, it may ignore the condition. I must remember to pause and respond, rather than react against pain. Take care of the injury or condition first and do not stop its acute pain. My response is to make sure the injury/condition is safe, its acute pain is no longer needed, and a doctor has said it is safe to control that pain before I control it.

The injury and pain are separate. Pain is not primary. Taking care of the injury is primary. Being prudent requires fully developed impulse and decision-making centers of the mind to resist temptations for stopping acute pain, and to objectively consider risks and consequences for appropriately applying CBi pain control techniques.

Given the need for a mature mind to determine when use is appropriate, children and teenagers' minds are not developed fully enough for them to exercise good judgment. Risks are too high for people under twenty.

Ten Precautions

1. Acute-like Chronic Pain

Making the pain go away does not mean you are in the clear or that you are cured. It may only mean you are very good at controlling pain. How well you control pain is not the most important thing. Your health is the most important thing. Heed any warning signs that a condition is getting worse, and act responsibly.

Whenever chronic pain has been silent for a while, but reawakens later, or the pain never went away entirely and is more painful now than before, that could indicate that the underlying condition has gotten worse. Consider any return of silenced pain to be acute, or any sudden, worsening change in the quality of previously controlled pain to now be acute. It's prudent to presume it's acute and has a valid purpose. Heed its warnings.

Treat chronic pain like acute pain if it becomes more painful. Perhaps the condition should be rediagnosed and a new decision should reached for dealing with a potentially worsening condition. Diagnosis takes priority. Feel the pain to obtain a proper, correct diagnosis.

Do not apply the Touch or MBPC techniques to new or changing pain. Do not ignore the messenger. Pay attention and heed pain's warning. Notice the pain, take mental or actual notes while the pain lasts, and take appropriate action. See a doctor. Allow the pain, so your doctor can witness it, through you, to reach a valid diagnosis. I repeat this because it's so important. It is often best to wait until your doctor tells you it is time to control the pain before applying CBi pain control techniques again.

2. Effects of CB Intrinsic Techniques

Controlling chronic pain does not mean you lose feeling. You do not become numb. It is like using pain pills, but unlike using pain pills, only the pain is affected. There is no fog nor are there risks for unwanted drug complications, dependence, abuses, or addiction. When the techniques have not been used for a while, and the body returns to baseline, acute pain will behave as it normally would, making itself known when necessary.

3. Full Effects Can Hide Acute Pain

While the powers of intrinsic techniques are in full force, and endorphins are active, injuries may go unnoticed and lie quietly in the shadows because acute pain may be inadvertently silenced with a higher pain threshold. You might see an infected sore on the back of your leg or notice an injury only because something looks and/or feels puffy. You may feel a hard lump under the skin, perhaps a painless pulled muscle. When you get a cut or scrape, you may only feel a twinge or mild tingling. Those are some signs of injury with a high pain threshold. Notice physical signs of infection, subtle sensations, and other changes that occur in the absence of actual pain. Become your own bodyguard.

If it is more difficult to feel acute pain now, due to a higher pain threshold, perform body scans periodically to search for unnoticed tissue damage. Visually scan yourself to see what could have been painful. Use mirrors to help you view hidden areas, for example, for checking the middle of your back. Being proactive is a good idea, and body checks only take a minute. It's good to not be hypersensitive to pain, but the bottom line is, if you see an infection and it doesn't hurt, get help anyway.

4. Pain Control Is Not a Cure

Remember that pain and the injury are separate. Pain control techniques do not necessarily cure the underlying condition, even if muscles or glands regain function. Be observant, be vigilant, check for signs of infection, worsening conditions, or new issues that need your attention. In the absence of pain, become your own alarm system.

5. Intrinsic Techniques with Minor Pain

Being able to control pain does not mean we should always do it. Be prudent. Acute pain should not be controlled until it has finished serving its purpose. I repeat that so often so knowing it becomes a part of you. But for those times we would use over-the-counter acetaminophen or aspirin for mild or minor pain, I usually try the Touch and MBPC first to see if they can be just as or more effective. I notice swelling from inflammation and treat that condition separately, allowing and monitoring its pain to judge its progress.

6. Take Strong Acute Pain Seriously

If chronic pain control is not running silently, globally in the background, you will clearly notice acute pain as it occurs. Strong acute pain with an undiagnosed condition should not be controlled. That pain must aid the diagnosis. Infection pain should never be controlled. That pain is necessary for gauging the infection's progress; pain lets us know whether the infection is getting better or worse. Even though it is fun to stop pain, we need to use common sense and refrain from controlling pain that still serves a vital purpose.

Acute Pain Exists to Assist.

7. Stubborn Acute or Chronic Pain

It may go without saying, but once acute pain becomes grizzly and grueling, and the emotional and physical drain from that condition becomes extreme, the condition is screaming angry because its status is critical. Before the emotional drain becomes extremely excessive or chronic pain suddenly resists control, make haste. The underlying condition may have seriously worsened. The landscape has changed. Check with your doctor. Perhaps surgery is nearly overdue.

As conditions worsen toward a critical turning point, surgical solutions or medical interventions may become more invasive or extreme to reach the same desired result. If pain prevents you from controlling it, don't delay. Allow the pain for a correct diagnosis and address the needs of the condition sooner than later.

Pain control is not the absolute goal. If the underlying condition becomes serious, being able to control pain is merely a preference, in comparison. Chronic pain that suddenly resists control may indicate the condition needs immediate attention or surgery. The focus must switch from a matter of pain control to taking care of a serious health issue.

Giving the best efforts to care for a condition, in a timely manner, is the primary goal. The window may close for receiving a less invasive cure. Health comes first. Be prudent. Don't postpone seeking a doctor's help.

8. Symptoms Other than Pain

Pain is not the only symptom alerting us to a very serious injury. There can also be nausea, grimacing, doubling over, and similar behaviors, as mentioned earlier. Pain control techniques do not affect those symptoms because they operate in different regions of the brain than pain does.

We can mistakenly believe that 'doubling over in pain' happens only because we are in so much pain; the 'pain made me' double over. While pain is being controlled, doubling over without the associated pain is startling, and eventually comical. The logical brain can't make sense of it. It is disorienting like an earthquake.

Once skilled in pain control techniques, you could experience this, so remember that doubling over is a definite sign of serious tissue damage or injury, even if it occurs without pain. These symptoms of serious injury become significant messengers for you to pay serious attention to, just as you would if your pain were being controlled with medication. Respond as you would have if very intense pain were accompanying the doubling-over, and get help soon.

9. Returning to Some Baseline

While MBPC and the Touch are in full effect, and endorphin pathways are turned on, your pain threshold for acute pain can rise, which causes you to not notice pain as much. Had you been hypersensitive to pain, hypersensitivity may be less of an issue.

Once chronic pain episodes have ended and normal acute pain processes are re-established, continuing to practice MBPC could improve health and wellness by mindfully reducing the ill-effects of long-term stress.

Pain control techniques might achieve full recovery from chronic pain by re-establishing normal, acute pain patterns, but at some point, pain control effects may wear off. Acute pain thresholds may drop, with pain becoming more noticeable again. An old condition might worsen to the point of becoming painful again. Do what shampoo bottles say to do. "Repeat." Allow the pain to get a diagnosis, seek treatment, and reapply the CBi techniques to control pain when appropriate. Easy.

10. Stop! Use Common Sense First!

Acute pain is here to help us; it is our friend. We can control inappropriate chronic pain as soon as we are certain it doesn't serve a purpose. We can control it. We can stop it. We even have neuroplasticity for potentially restoring normal acute pain processing. Using the techniques appropriately allows me to genuinely appreciate pain, rather than fear it. That's fine except, the mind makes us think that controlling pain is primary.

When it is pointed out, adults easily recognize that our primary goal is to optimize health, rather than only control pain. Yet young minds think that stopping pain is all that counts. It is wise to not teach these techniques to children or teenagers because stopping every pain is a temptation with hidden, serious consequences. When it isn't pointed out, even adults find it difficult to stop themselves from using chronic pain control techniques without first considering priorities and potential, unintended, negative consequences. Even I have used poor judgment.

Common sense has a habit of waiting until something dawns on us before we notice it. For example, I began making potentially serious mistakes in 2012 with my new techniques because I didn't pause to consider risks first. I was lucky not to suffer permanent, negative consequences. These near misses got my attention and reinforced the fact that I need to strongly warn against inappropriately controlling certain types of pain.

I discovered that applying MBPC techniques alone can reduce or stop the pain of wasp stings. I didn't use the Touch because the wasp stung me on my back where I couldn't reach it. Applying MBPC techniques that first time took about two minutes to absolutely stop the pain, and the stinging pain never returned. I was amazed. As unexpectedly, when I checked the sting on my back, the infection I saw from the sting's puncture wound didn't hurt either. I took appropriate action and went to the doctor for treatment to take care of the 'painless' infection from the wasp sting. That was common sense.

A month or two later, I received three stings from a hornet. I realized I had been stung only after I shooed the hornet away from my arm and saw that it left three small, rectangular welts. Reflecting on it, I realized I felt slight electric buzzes, which might have been stings, but they were more like tickles. Apparently, my brain learned from my earlier wasp sting to automatically prevent new stings from creating pain. I am frequently stung, and noticed that it took over a year for my desensitization to stings to wear off enough for me to feel a sting again.

Then it dawned on me in 2017, as I disturbed a wasp nest in a pile of leaves, that our caliber of common sense matters. Don't use common sense like I know, I know. This common sense must be intelligent common sense.

I didn't notice those wasps in 2017 until I felt two simultaneous stings – one on my hand and the other on my back. I flicked the wasp off of my hand and concentrated on stopping the pains, as I received the third sting, again on my back. It took me about 15 or 20 seconds to silence all three sting pains via MBPC alone.

I looked up and saw I was surrounded by a tall column of angry wasps. It's amazing how calm I had become around wasps. While they used to terrify me, taking away the pain of their sting removed my fear of them. I needed to keep working with the leaves, so I ignored the wasps. I later counted 8 painless stings.

Since I was only focusing on stopping pain, it didn't dawn on me that my common sense was too 'common.' I had to educate myself about wasp venom. Wasp venom causes our immune system to become allergic to it. Getting more stings equals having more venom, which eventually causes a permanent, life threatening allergy to venom. I could imagine a cartoon character saying, "It's not about the pain silly. It's the venom! Run!"

My mind tricked me for years into commonly believing that stopping the acute stinging pain was primary. I was wrong. Since exposure to venom is a ticking time bomb, avoiding wasp, hornet or bee sting venom is the primary goal. We must become educated about our current situation or condition to raise the quality of our common sense in order to use pain control intelligently and wisely.

Pain is only the messenger. While I silenced the messenger, I was ignorant of the true threat. While silencing the pain, I should have run away, regardless of how trivial I considered a swarm of wasps, and regardless of how important I thought continuing my task was. Learn from my mistakes.

Remember that unless chronic pain is the condition, stopping pain is not the priority. Remember that taking care of the condition and protecting function always matters most. Be prudent by being correct. Become educated about your situation so your common sense of the highest quality. Consult with a doctor to help make certain you are correct. Set priorities first and only take risks you can afford to lose and not regret.

Applying all of those considerations, we would think that retired football players with arthritis or football players recovering from surgery could benefit greatly from using pain control techniques. On the other hand, someone might injure a leg during a school football game, control the pain with CBi techniques, feel no pain, regain muscle function as if nothing had happened, and then go back out onto the field to play right away. An adult can see that is obviously not a good idea. Let's also consider how it's not so obvious to a child or teenager.

The stage of brain development is what distinguishes children and teenagers from adults. Young brains lack self-control against temptation, the ability to be prudent, the ability to exercise educated, quality common sense, or to recognize the vital need for allowing acute pain.

It's quality common sense that we should not even apply the Touch to children, except for a mother's gentle, light kiss, until they have become adults before learning these skills (terminal illnesses exempted).

Always remember that controlling pain does not need to be primary. MBPC allows us to lessen the intensity and urgency of pain without needing to stop it. We can appreciate the hidden, yet lifesaving significance and value of allowing acute pain to exist in order to use it as intended - an incentive and mechanism for protecting the injury from further harm, a force for taking appropriate action, an alarm for gauging whether a condition is getting better or worse, and its essential role for obtaining a correct diagnosis.

A Few Limitations

CBi Touch and MBPC techniques do come with some imperfections. Wouldn't it be perfect if we could tell pain to stop and it would? Masters at CBi Touch and MBPC can do that. Perfect would be even better if, after controlling pain, we could ask our body to turn the right kind of pain on again for a few moments to help us see how the condition is doing. Sometimes that happens, but unfortunately, we can't will pain to turn on again, even with these techniques. Whether or when the pain returns is fairly random. There are other limitations.

1. Adults Only - Not Children or Teenagers

Mature minds are required for safe application of pain control techniques. It isn't that children would not be able to learn the techniques and apply them. The problem is that children would learn the techniques and apply them inappropriately, due to lack of self-control.

Children cannot imagine the dangers inherent in stopping a pain that still serves a purpose and would apply the Touch if an adult were not watching. Imagine being young and told not to control searing pain. Youth would ignore that advice and stop their pain, rather than being tortured by it. They can't fear the danger enough.

Still apply the kiss to your child's scratched knee, but do not disclose its secret. Young people benefit from mindfulness techniques to reduce hypersensitivity to pain and lower stress levels in general, but it is too dangerous to teach them intrinsic techniques that actually stop pain.

Pain control techniques are for adults only. One of my doctors suggests that waiting until an adult has matures, is perhaps 25 years old, would be a good idea.

Pain serves a vital purpose. Pain teaches vital lessons. Children and teens learn from it. Consider these techniques a luxury that requires maturity and self-control. Make this accessible only to capable adults.

2. Easy to Reach

The Touch is easier to apply when an injury is easy to reach; head, lower back, abdomen, arms, hips, knees, and legs may be easy. Yet, it is impossible for your hands to apply the Touch to pinched spinal nerve pain located between your shoulder blades. In cases like that, a feather duster makes it easy to deliver a light touch. Asking a friend or family member willing to apply the Touch for you might also help. In a pinch, a neighbor may be happy to help. Sharing this information with your neighbors may even help them. Win-Win

3. Chronic Conditions

Conditions for which acute pains continually renew are less likely to be helped by the Touch, or at least right away. MBPC works best for those situations. The Touch would also not be able to help if the touch neurons in the skin have been permanently damaged or are impaired.

4. Inadvertent Inappropriate Use

Limitations for the Touch must obviously warn against inappropriately stopping acute pain before its purpose has been served. We occasionally and inadvertently apply the Touch without realizing it. Children want their mommy to lightly kiss the new scratch on their knee because it makes the pain go away. Notice how often something lightly brushes across your skin, just in passing. Notice how often pain stops seemingly for no reason, spontaneously. Was there truly no reason, or did a soft touch go unnoticed? A very soft touch can fight pain, whether we intended it to or not.

5. Hidden Automatic Effects

Unlike the Touch, MBPC applies to the whole body and can become automatic, given my experiences it.

For MBPC to work, one must remain awake long enough for it to take full effect. One must have functional neural pain control pathways in the brain, brainstem, and spinal cord. Pain control pathways that have abnormally wired themselves (chronic pain) are still 'functional'. MBPC helps those abnormalities rewire to unlearn chronic pain and re-establish normal pain pathways, through neuroplasticity.

People display a full range of sensitivities to pain and MBPC can raise basically anyone's pain threshold, meaning it takes more injury to cause the same amount of pain. With a higher pain threshold, one becomes less sensitive to painful stimulus. Therefore, with the help of MBPC, the pain may not feel as intense as it used to. As with others who are not hypersensitive to pain, do not wait for extreme pain before judging a condition's severity. Be observant and use common sense.

6. Opioid Interference

Following anesthesia or with opioids on board for a short period of time, as might be the case during surgery recovery, the Touch may take between a moment or a couple of minutes to work. If the Touch does not relieve surgery recovery pain, try again after the anesthesia and medications have time to wear off. Sometimes, short-term narcotics use doesn't interfere at all, but that depends on the individual, and many other variables.

Following a long-term narcotic painkiller regimen for months to years, the Touch may or may not be effective, again depending on many variables. The longer the exposure to narcotic painkillers, the longer it may take the Touch to work, even to the point of not working for some. It has been easier for the Touch to work for those individuals after drug treatment is finished, and the nervous system has had time to recover from the long-term, negative impacts of opioids. Everyone is different.

7. Inflammation

The Touch and MBPC can sometimes stop inflammation pain, but pain control is neither cure nor remedy for the condition of inflammation. Remember that pain is only the messenger. Inflammation is an immune system process that can be toxic and chronic. Treat it as a separate threat because it damages and erodes good tissues, including nervous tissue, over time. Seek your doctor's help to effectively control it. Addressing and minimizing inflammation is a major part of controlling chronic pain effectively.

Notes

NBC Nightly News reporter Dr. John Torres featured the surprising virtual reality (VR) study results from Stanford Neuropsychiatrist, Dr. Kim Bullock. The studies used VR treatments to relieve patients' anxiety, but patients also experienced relief from chronic pain symptoms, lasting from weeks to months. One of Dr. Bullock's patients, Pierre Martineau, was featured. He suffered chronic pain with muscle weakness in his injured arm. After five weekly VR treatments with Dr. Bullock, Pierre's pain disappeared, as his muscle function improved to nearly normal. Pain expert Dr. Sean Mackey, who was also featured from Stanford, said that VR tricks the brain into normalizing pain.[1]

The CBi Touch from the bottom-up and Mindfulness-based Pain Control (MBPC) techniques from the top-down share common outcomes with VR results. They all trick the nervous system into normalizing various pain stopping pathways to alleviate chronic pain and improve muscle function.

May 28, 2020

Completing this third edition of my book fulfills the purpose of my pain control journey. It gives value to my conditions that have caused so much pain. It gives purpose to my education in neurobiology and the other sciences. May this book reach and help others I could not help otherwise. And may referring back to the book make practicing and finding success with MBPC easier.

---

[1] Torres, J. (Reporter), & Snow, K. (Anchor). (2017, May 28). Can Virtual Reality Sessions Treat Chronic Pain? [Television series episode]. NBC Nightly News. Retrieved from https://archives.nbclearn.com/portal/site/k-12/browse/?cuecard=111791 and https://www.youtube.com/watch?v=FOTGlD5HC1A

June 14, 2020

Rest assured that the CBi Touch and Mindfulness-based Pain Control techniques are evidence and science based, even though they are extraordinary and offer revolutionary ways to control pain with minimal or no reliance on pain meds. The principles behind CBi pain control techniques (the Touch and MBPC) are supported by many times the nearly 500 peer-reviewed, scientific journal articles I have collected over the past several years. Understanding these findings from cognitive neuroscience and neurobiology research can help practitioners and patients alike grasp how this is possible.

Those scientific findings help explain why and how the Touch and the MBPC techniques effectively trick the nervous system into unlearning chronic pain, re-establishing normal pain processing pathways, and sometimes aid in regaining muscle and/or gland functions, depending on the condition.

Integrating those research findings, while explaining the science itself, so the how's and why's will make sense to those unfamiliar with it, will be a massive undertaking. I intend to write both a generalized book for the scientifically curious, and its fraternal twin, a detailed textbook on pain and pain control for health and wellness schools, massage and physical therapists, and healthcare practitioners in general.

Pain control is a beneficial part of us. As injuries heal, it is natural and normal for our nervous system to intrinsically stop creating their pains. As long as adults heed the warnings about the known limitations and precautions that go along with controlling pain intrinsically, never use it to control infection pain, only control pain for diagnosed conditions and with their doctor's permission, remember that the pain and its condition are separate, and prioritize health, function, and treating the condition over controlling its pain, they can learn how to manipulate their nervous system to reap the benefits of appropriately applied pain control. Through MBPC, they can also reduce the ill effects prolonged stress forces on the mind, the immune system, organ health, and body systems. Mindfulness practices, including MBPC techniques, are so healthy because they hamper the ability of long-term stress to create illnesses and diseases over time.

CBi pain control techniques provide intrinsic alternatives and enhance pain management. Respond rather than react to pain, change your relationship with pain, claim its power for yourself, redefine your reality about pain, improve your health, and start reclaiming your life. We are meant to live life lusciously, intrinsically, from within.

Made in the USA
San Bernardino, CA
22 June 2020

73877461R00158